NAS

NURSES' AIDS SERIES

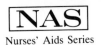

Nurses' Aids Series

THEATRE NURSING

Technique and Care

Sixth Edition

Bernice J.M. West, MA (Hons), RGN
Nursing Development Officer
Nursing Development Unit
City Hospital and Foresterhill College of Nursing,
Aberdeen

BAILLIERE TINDALL
London Philadelphia Toronto Sydney Tokyo

Baillière Tindall 24–28 Oval Road,
W.B. Saunders London NW1 7DX

The Curtis Center,
Independence Square West,
Philadelphia, PA 19106–3399, USA

55 Horner Avenue,
Toronto, Ontario M8Z 4X6, Canada

Harcourt Brace Jovanovich (Australia) Pty Ltd,
32–52 Smidmore Street,
Marrickville, NSW 2204, Australia

Harcourt Brace Jovanovich Japan Inc.,
Ichibancho Central Building, 22–1 Ichibancho,
Chiyoda-ku, Tokyo 102, Japan

© 1992 Baillière Tindall

First published 1944
Fourth edition 1967
 Reprinted 1971, 1973, 1974, 1975, 1978, 1979, 1981
Fifth edition 1983
 Reprinted 1987
Sixth edition 1992

ISBN 0 7020 1605 5

Spanish edition (CECSA Barcelona) 1967
Turkish edition (Turkish Government) 1960

A catalogue record for this book is available from the British Library.

Typeset by Photo·graphics, Honiton, Devon
Printed in England by Clays Ltd, St Ives plc

Contents

Acknowledgements

A textbook such as this evolves from discussions with many people. I am indebted to the nursing and medical staff of G1–G8 theatres, Aberdeen Royal Infirmary, who taught me in the first instance and who supported me as a teacher and researcher within the operating department.

The Education Sub-committee of the National Association of Theatre Nurses deserves special thanks, as do my other colleagues in the Association. Many of the ideas presented have been clarified and developed through the work of NATN.

Sarah Smith of Baillière Tindall has not only been an editor but also a friend during the production of the text. Grateful acknowledgement is also made to Eileen Dixon, the author of the previous edition of *Theatre Technique*, and the various firms who supplied photographs.

Finally, it would have been impossible to produce the text without the love, support and guidance of Michael Lyon, the love of my life.

Bernice J.M. West
January 1992

Preface

Developments in surgical nursing have occurred in their multitudes over the last decade. Since the publication of the last edition of *Theatre Technique* there has been a major trend in nursing towards patient-centred care. Nurses have become concerned with standard-setting, patient advocacy and professional autonomy. New educational curricula have been introduced for nurses, operating department assistants and support workers. On the technical front, laser surgery has advanced and become popular, as has day-case surgery. Operations which previously required a patient to be hospitalised for a week are now conducted on a day-case basis.

Developments in anaesthetic drugs, monitoring techniques, endoscopic equipment, stapling devices, *in vitro* fertilisation techniques and life support measures have all occurred.

Consumer Protection and Data Protection Acts have come into being, as has the computerisation of theatre management and stock systems. Patient charters, hospital trusts and business plans are now common parlance in health-care provision, and the operating department is focal in acute-sector care.

On a sadder note, we have seen the advent of HIV and AIDS amongst the population, and the implications of these diseases for theatre workers must not be underestimated.

This book will not try to analyse and present an account

of all these developments, but, rather, its aims are similar to those in the original *Theatre Technique*; namely, to provide clear and concise information for the theatre nurse or operating department assistant.

Some of the excellent illustrations from the last edition have been retained, but the text has been largely re-written and re-sequenced in order to present an analysis of peri-operative nursing.

Finally, each chapter may be read independently, and further reading is recommended. Some chapters conclude with an exercise, which can be carried out as a group discussion or by self-reflective study.

Bernice J.M. West

Introduction

The major recommendations contained within recent government white papers, new curricula for nurse education and new training for operating department assistants offer many challenges for theatre nursing within the United Kingdom.

All students must be provided with the appropriate experience to ensure that they have a full understanding of pre-, intra- and post-operative nursing care. Patient care does not only occur in a ward or in the community. A great deal of nursing care is carried out in specialist departments where technical skills are required in addition to conventional nursing skills. For these reasons it is important to incorporate nursing care in the operating department into the student nurse educational curricula.

As the operating department is totally new as an environment and as a learning situation from the point of view of all students, there can be little doubt that without associated instruction the theatre experience could be a waste of time. It is essential that the student's time in theatre is relevant to the nursing care of the surgical patient. This book aims to provide an insight into the care of the surgical patient and specific techniques essential to nursing in the operating department.

Students may spend a clear period of time in the operating department or may visit on a daily basis with specific patients. It is important to ensure that any time spent is seen as beneficial, as this will affect recruitment of staff into the operating department in the future. This new text focuses on peri-operative nursing care, and will be of value to the student who spends a day in the operating department, to the trainee operating department assistant or to the newly qualified nurse who plans to specialise in theatre nursing.

NURSING IN THE OPERATING DEPARTMENT

Over the last twenty years the role of the nurse in the operating department has been publicly questioned through official reports and research projects. In order to identify clearly the role of the nurse in the operating department official reports in 1970 and later in 1990 stated that new grades of theatre staff should be introduced. These new grades would focus on the technical aspects of theatre work and thereby enable the nurse to carry out pure nursing duties.

Several authors have called for one grade of theatre worker in order to standardise the training and career opportunities for all grades of staff. Others have suggested that theatre nurses should be involved in total patient care and develop unique nursing skills within the operating department.

The failure to make proper use of nursing 'skills' in operating departments, which had been observed, has been remedied in a few areas in recent years. However, a general dissatisfaction amongst theatre nurses has been identified in many research studies. Early studies carried out from the mid-1960s onwards have ascertained that problems exist in both retaining and recruiting nurses into the operating department. Two main reasons are usually given: firstly, morale is generally low due to excessive working hours and standby duties; secondly, nearly a third of nursing time was estimated to be spent on non-nursing tasks.

Recent research has shown that, although more ancillary and technical workers have been employed in operating departments, the reasons for job dissatisfaction amongst nurses remain the same as they were before. Lack of patient contact and development of nursing care have been identified as contributing to wastage and recruitment problems. In order to combat these problems and also to utilise more fully theatre nurses' skills, care plans have been designed for theatre use. Further, these projects have all involved theatre nurses visiting patients pre-operatively and post-operatively. Research concludes that both the patient and the nurse benefit from pre- and post-operative visiting.

Health promotion

The educative role of the nurse in the pre-operative situation was first identified through systematic research in 1975. This research showed that, when appropriate information about pain expectations was given to patients pre-operatively, their experiences of anxiety and pain were reported as reduced post-operatively. Following on from this study, another researcher in 1978 concluded that when information is given to patients prior to surgery, their recovery is enhanced.

Theatre nurse researchers have identified the role of the theatre nurse as critical in reducing post-operative pain and anxiety by visiting surgical patients. Consequently, the role of the theatre nurse has been extended recently to include a closer liaison with ward staff and communication with surgical patients.

1 Pre-operative nursing care in the operating department

Working in the operating department offers the nurse a unique opportunity to participate in the total care of patients requiring surgery. Whilst in the department the nurse can expect to participate as a member of a highly skilled, multi-disciplinary team committed to peri-operative care.

In the operating department the comprehensive, pre-operative care of the surgical patient is essential. This involves:

1. Assessing the physical and psychological well-being of surgical patients through pre-operative interviewing.
2. Planning, implementing and evaluating appropriate care.
3. Documenting patient needs and nursing actions.
4. Educating and supporting parents or significant others.
5. Preparing equipment for the safe care of the patient during various types of anaesthesia or sedation.
6. Communicating effectively in order to reduce patient anxiety and to promote good working relationships within the multi-disciplinary team.
7. Identifying and acting upon potential hazards to both patients and staff and, where appropriate, acting to prevent injury.

8. Identifying potential complications of various anaesthetic or sedative drugs.
9. Recognising the early signs of complications and acting upon these as appropriate.

These objectives cover the entire pre-operative preparation of the patient. In order to appreciate the value of the objectives and their wider implications, this section will focus on the psychology of surgery and pre-operative visiting.

PSYCHOLOGICAL REACTIONS TO SURGERY

Self-image

The term 'self-image' refers to the highly personal view each of us has of ourselves. This includes our physical image, but it is much broader in that it includes the general way we feel and think about ourselves. An individual person is not born with a self-image, but, rather, it develops and is substantially derived from our interactions with other people (Price, 1990).

Generally speaking, if individuals obtain positive messages about themselves they will internalise these perceptions and develop a positive self-image. If, however, they receive negative messages from other people, then they may come to see themselves in negative terms.

Most patients have a reasonably positive self-image most of the time, but when illness or change in body appearance occurs they may begin to question certain previously held assumptions about themselves. When this happens it is important that the nurse can plan nursing care and interventions in such a way as to enable the individual to accept these changes.

Independence and self-control

Although each person's self-image is idiosyncratic, in any particular culture there are often common elements. Two concepts for nurses to consider when caring for patients whose self-image has been altered or damaged due to surgical intervention are independence and self-control.

Most people recognise that independence and dependency are interrelated. Each person has a need for other people, and yet, at the same time, each of us also has the ability to do without others for long periods of time.

For those who place special value on independence the prospect of relying on someone else is daunting. For such patients the worst fear is that, by receiving help from the nurse, they may become completely dependent on the nurse. To help alleviate this feeling state, it is important that nurses include patients in any decision-making process. By accepting and respecting the individual's concern for independence and self-control, nursing help will be accepted to a limited degree by all patients.

Virtually the opposite of the very independent person are those who see themselves as having very little self-control or self-determination. Some people feel that things just happen to them, and they believe that other people actually determine life-events for them. Such patients may want the nurse to take control, and the idea that they themselves could influence personal problems and difficulties may seem implausible. In fact, the individual may be afraid of taking control because of an absence of resources and ability to care for this new self-image. The nurse must introduce the patient to self-control in a very gradual manner and not rush in with false reassurance (Price, 1990).

Grieving

Whilst the range of factors affecting personal response to surgery is extensive, most research into this topic by nurses and social scientists has characterised the response in terms of grieving. The grief reaction is believed to occur in response to lost body attributes, attractiveness and body presentation. This grieving process has been analysed as progressing through a number of stages.

Stage 1 *Shock*: At this stage the patient cannot comprehend what is about to happen or has happened, and is not as capable as usual of making decisions.

Stage 2 *Denial*: The patient wishes to deny the facts, or the events that are happening, and may appear to the nurse to be unconcerned about the surgery.

Stage 3 *Anger*: Patients are usually very angry about what has happened to themselves at this stage, and may direct the anger to the nurse or internalise the feelings and become withdrawn.

Stage 4 *Depression*: At this stage patients may have internalised their feelings to such an extent that depression ensues and hope is lost.

Stage 5 *Bargaining*: Patients begin to compromise or bargain with themselves, family and nursing staff in order to try and accept the implications of the surgery.

Stage 6 *Acceptance*: The patient has now accepted

and become reconciled to the outcome.

These stages have been drawn from Kübler-Ross's work (1969) with the terminally ill and their families. The stages identified are not necessarily linear, and patients may linger in, or return to, earlier stages. This model helps understanding of the psychological processes that many surgical patients experience, especially those patients who have undergone extensive and mutilating surgery.

It is necessary to remember, however, that not all patients will perceive their surgery and subsequent altered body image as undesirable. Some patients will even welcome it as a sign of new status. The recognition of the alteration may relieve the patient of previously onerous responsibilities and stresses.

The nurse must realise that the personal response of the surgical patient is the definition of that new identity. In order to understand this it is necessary for the nurse to support or enable this new identity to be negotiated, through interactions between the patient and others.

To assist with this process the theatre nurse may wish to contribute to a patient self-help group which may exist at ward level. Alternatively, during a pre-operative interview the nurse may inform the patient that he or she will participate in a post-operative interview aimed at assisting the patient with the outcome of the surgery.

PRE-OPERATIVE VISITING AND INTERVIEWING

The patient pre-operative visit and interview is a complex process which requires good communication skills and sound clinical knowledge. By careful interviewing the nurse can obtain relevant information from patients in order to plan more individual and effective care.

The purpose of the pre-operative interview is to elicit meaningful information from the patient in order that care can be planned systematically in the operating department. In order to do this effectively trust and empathy must be built up.

Interviewing skills

Whilst observing and interviewing the patient, it is essential that the nurse is aware of verbal and non-verbal communication cues coming from each party. For very often the verbal account tells one story and the body posture another. Good eye contact is necessary if the nurse is to build up trust with the patient. It is important for the nurse to pay particular attention to the duration of eye contact, as staring can be intimidating. The occasional smile and nod encourages replies, and shows the patient that you are listening and affirms what the patient is saying.

It will also help easy communication if the nurse faces the patient and leans forward slightly in order to encourage openness, interest and trust.

When speaking with the patient, the nurse should avoid halting speech, and other paralinguistic idiosyncrasies, such as the use of 'OK'. The use of normal, everyday English expressions rather than technical terms, and the modification of dialect and accent to suit the patient encourages and facilitates dialogue.

Interview technique

Before conducting the pre-operative interview it is useful to have prepared a check-list of questions pertinent to the care of the particular patient being interviewed. It is essential that the patient consents to be interviewed.

The language chosen for the interview is important.

Emotionally charged or emotive words are best avoided. It the patient is reluctant to answer a particular range of questions, avoid over-emphasising this topic as the patient will become anxious. Forcing answers from patients is not acceptable. The most meaningful information can be elicited from patients using non-directive techniques. To clarify what the patient has said it is often useful to repeat what has been said in the form of a question, using the patient's own words rather than technical terms. Sometimes it is useful to disclose personal feelings and experiences, as this often enables the patient to share openly.

Finally, it is necessary to ask only one question at a time and listen carefully to the answer. If too many questions are asked that begin with the word 'why', patients may feel that their personal values are being questioned.

Interview structure

For effective communication to take place a social introduction is necessary. This can easily be achieved by the theatre nurse telling the patient his or her name and title. As with any interview situation, pre-surgical patients will respond better when informed of what is expected of them. Therefore during the introduction it is often beneficial to inform the patient

- why the interview is being carried out,
- in what ways this interview is different from others,
- how it will help the patient's care in the operating department.

The timing of the interview is important for both parties. By carefully selecting a time for the pre-operative interview that is suitable to both and by careful pre-

Table 1.1

HOSPITAL NAME & ADDRESS

Pre-operative visiting form

Surname .... Forename .... Mrs/Mr/Miss

Male/Female ....

Date of birth .... Hospital number ....

Ward .... Consultant .... Date of admission ....

Diagnosis .... Proposed operation ....

Date of pre-operative visit ....

<u>Brief summary of illness leading to admission</u>

This information can be retrieved from the notes

<u>Observations</u> (please circle)

tall/medium height/short
obese/average weight for height/thin
glasses/contact lenses/dentures/hearing aid

Other prostheses (please state)

Spoken language ....

Any language or speech difficulties? ....

<u>Present health problems as seen by the patient</u>

Brief summary

<u>Emotional state</u>   cheerful/calm/anxious/distressed/
unresponsive

Have you been in hospital before? yes/no
Have you had previous surgery? yes/no
If yes, what was the operation?

Table 1.2

Has the doctor given you all the information you want to know? yes/no

Comments

What have the ward staff told you about your preparation for theatre?
Brief details

Check that the patient is aware of the following:
1. The importance of pre-operative fasting
2. The reasons for:
   a. Wearing theatre gown and cap
   b. Removing jewellery, prostheses, make-up and hairclips
   c. Remaining in bed after the administration of premedication
   d. Other pre-operative preparations, e.g. enema, bowel preparation

Have you got any joint conditions or diseases that limit movement?
yes/no
Comment if necessary

Have you got any allergies? yes/no
Comment if necessary

Are there any questions you would like to ask me?
(Be prepared to listen and comment here, if necessary.)

Visiting nurse's signature ....

General comments on the use of this form

The examining doctor will have charted relevant clinical details and it is not deemed necessary to subject the patient to unnecessary questioning again. The role of the visiting nurse is to make written relevant observations on which the nursing objectives will be based and to assist the patient in coming to terms with the impending surgery. No promise should be given regarding the outcome of surgery, but it would be encouraging to the patient if arrangements are made (with him) to visit him post-operatively.

interview preparation by the nurse, repetition of information can be avoided and disturbances minimised. The physical and emotional comfort of the patient is essential. Privacy assists here, as does recapitulation of the information given which in turn enables the patient to feel involved in the care being planned.

Topic for discussion

Consider the value of the information sheet below, which has been prepared for patients. What information has been omitted? How useful are standardised information leaflets?

What happens in the operating theatre?

This is a question many patients ask themselves before and after an operation.

There are many nurses who choose to work in the highly skilled and demanding area of the operating theatre. Before they come to work in theatres, all nurses have undergone a general training programme which lasts for either two or three years. In addition, many nurses have also undertaken courses to enhance their specialist knowledge of surgery, anaesthetics and post-operative patient care.

If you have been to theatre before you will know that the nurses who work there wear green pyjama suits rather than white uniforms. This is for comfort and cleanliness.

Whilst in the operating department, as a patient, you will be cared for by a nurse at all times. The nurse will plan your care from the time you arrive at the department until the time you leave to return to the ward.

When you first arrive in the department you will be transferred into the anaesthetic room. This room has a wide variety of equipment – but don't be alarmed. For the nurse, the operating department assistant and the anaesthetist these are the routine and essential pieces of equipment to enable them to do their job. A nurse will be with you whilst you receive your anaesthetic, and will then accompany you into the operating theatre and stay with you and the anaesthetist for the operation.

Whilst you have been in the anaesthetic room other nurses

have been preparing the equipment for your operation and setting up the operating theatre. The nurse who prepared the surgical instruments will then assist during your operation – working closely with the doctors to care for you.

Other nurses will also be present in theatre to care for you safely, monitor what is happening, check swabs and instruments and provide any extra equipment required during your operation. When your operation is over a nurse will accompany you to the recovery room of the theatre where you will wake up from your anaesthetic. In the recovery room you will be looked after by a nurse until you are ready to return to your ward.

FURTHER READING

Boore, J. (1978) *Prescription for Recovery*, RCN, London.

Boore, J. (1980) *Pre-operative Information and Post-operative Recovery*, RCN, London.

Cox, H. (1987) 'The peri-operative role – a personal view', *Natnews* (Jan.), pp. 15–16.

Farmer, G. (1985) 'The role of the anaesthetic nurse', *Natnews* (Nov.), pp. 10–12.

Gooch, J. (1984) *The Other Side of Surgery*, Macmillan, Basingstoke.*

Gruendemann, B.J. *et al.* (1977) *The Surgical Patient – Behavioral Concepts for the Operating Room Nurse*, Mosby, St Louis, MO.

Hamilton-Smith, S. (1972) *Nil by Mouth*, RCN Research Series 1, No. 1, London.

Hayward, J. (1974) *Information – a Prescription against Pain*, RCN, London.*

Higgins, N. (1985) 'The case for pre-operative visiting', *Natnews* (March), p. 21.

Kalideen, D.P. and Leonard, M.D. (1985) 'So you're going to have an operation', *Natnews* (Feb.), pp. 12–21.*

Kübler-Ross, E. (1969) *On Death and Dying*, Macmillan, New York.

MDU, MPS, MDDUS, NATN, RCN (1986) *Theatre Safeguards*.

NATN (1991) *Principles of Safe Practice in the Operating Department – a Resource Book*, NATN, Harrogate, Yorkshire.*

Nightingale, K. (1987) *Learning to Care in the Theatre*, Hodder & Stoughton, London.*

Price, B. (1990) *Body Image*, Prentice Hall, London.

Warren, M. (1978) 'The receiving nurse in the operating theatre', *Natnews* (Nov.), p. 10.

---

* Highly recommended

Warren, M. (1981) 'The total care of a patient within the operating theatre', *Natnews*, 1,814, pp. 13–15.
Warren, M. (1983) *Operating Theatre Nursing*, Harper & Row, London.

2 Anaesthesia

PREPARATION FOR ANAESTHESIA

In the twentieth century much progress has been made
in anaesthesia, and since the 1950s the techniques of
anaesthesia and the drugs used have evolved rapidly.
Sophisticated equipment allows the anaesthetist to monitor the patient's bodily systems with a high degree of
accuracy, and the wide range of anaesthetic agents
available should ensure that each patient is given a
safe, satisfactory anaesthetic with minimal side-effects.
Anaesthesia is now recognised as a special branch of
medicine and nursing. Nurses working in this area should
have the knowledge and skills to care for the patient with
competence and compassion.

The anaesthetist visits the patient pre-operatively in
order to assess his fitness for anaesthesia and it is the
anaesthetist's responsibility to state whether or not the
patient is fit for operation. This applies particularly to
patients for elective surgery, which may not be immediately necessary. If the anaesthetist discovers any pre-
existing medical condition in the patient's physical state
which may complicate the operation, he may advise that
treatment be arranged to rectify this before surgery is
carried out. Careful physical assessment of the patient
requiring emergency surgery is essential, but when speed
is the most important consideration, the skill of the
anaesthetist and the selection of technique are also
significant factors.

Psychological preparation will facilitate the patient's adjustment to impending surgery: the ward and theatre staff can help considerably in this. Pre-operative visiting by an experienced theatre nurse helps to reassure the patient and lessens anxiety.

Consent

It is the surgeon's responsibility to explain the proposed operation and its possible outcome, and when he is satisfied that the patient understands, he will request the patient to sign a consent form. This is *solely* the duty of the surgeon, or one of his team, and must never be undertaken by nursing staff. Strict guidelines regarding consent to surgery and anaesthesia are laid down by the Medical Defence Union, the National Association of Theatre Nurses and the Royal College of Nursing, and these should be firmly adhered to.

Premedication

The purpose of premedication is twofold:

1. To depress vagus activity by drying up secretions,
2. To reduce anxiety.

Premedication is usually given at least one hour before the operation. This ensures that the patient is calm and sleepy on arrival in the theatre.

RECEPTION OF THE PATIENT

The patient's identity, the operation site and the consent form are checked by the anaesthetist prior to administering any anaesthetic drugs. It is important that noise levels are kept to a minimum in the anaesthetic room and that all equipment is prepared in advance. The surgeon or his deputy will consult with the patient prior to surgery. The nurse should check that all relevant notes and radiographs have accompanied the patient to the operating department. The patient's dentures and jewellery will have been removed by ward staff. Other prostheses may accompany the patient. It is therefore essential that these are stored safely and returned to the patient on recovery from anaesthesia. Subtle make-up can help to improve a patient's morale, but it may obscure vital signs, such as skin-colour, and for this reason it should not be worn. A register of all patients entering the operating theatre must be maintained: the patient's details are entered by the nurse delivering the patient. The final entry, giving the details of the operation performed, the surgeon's and anaesthetist's names and the nursing staff involved, are entered by the 'scrubbed' nurse or operating department assistant.

PREPARATION

Once induction of anaesthesia is complete, all the necessary equipment for the selected anaesthetic procedure and for positioning the patient should be readily at hand. Delays at this stage can pass on through the entire procedure and can endanger the patient or impair the surgeon's plan of operation.

Before any anaesthetic is commenced, certain basic essentials should be to hand:

(a) An efficient suction apparatus in working order, and a variety of suction catheters.

(b) The patient should be lying on a trolley or operating table which can be tipped head-down.

(c) In emergency cases, stomach tubes may be required to remove liquid gastric contents before starting induction. A suitable range of such tubes should be available.

(d) Resuscitation equipment should be available.
(e) The apparatus and drugs for the specific anaesthetic should be at hand.

INDUCTION

Anaesthesia may be induced by:

1. Intravenous injection
2. Inhalation
3. Local anaesthetic technique.

Intravenous injection

Intravenous injection is the most commonly used method of inducing anaesthesia. The drugs are usually given in a dose sufficient to produce light sleep.

Inhalation agents

Agents used include nitrous oxide, a compressed gas, isofluorane and halothane, which are all volatile liquids.

Local anaesthetics

Local anaesthetics are used as an alternative to general anaesthetics, as a supplement to general anaesthetic or as a technique for pain-relief post-operatively.

With local anaesthetic techniques, as for spinal and epidural anaesthesia, the patient often remains awake throughout the procedure. The rest of the team must be informed, so that undue noise is prevented; the patient must be cared for by a nurse throughout the operation to give assurance, comfort the patient and alleviate anxiety.

SPINAL AND EPIDURAL ANAESTHESIA

Spinal anaesthesia is produced by injecting a solution of local anaesthetic into the cerebrospinal fluid through a lumbar puncture needle so that it bathes a portion of the spinal cord and associated nerve roots. This renders part of the body analgesic and may paralyse the muscles. Depending on the volume and density of the solution and the position of the patient, the extent of analgesia can be controlled.

Epidural anaesthesia entails the injection of a comparatively large volume of local anaesthetic solution into the space outside the dura, thus affecting the nerves as they traverse the extradural space to escape from the vertebral column. The volume of solution and position of the patient determines the extent of the effect.

Both techniques cause a fall in blood pressure if the drugs reach thoracic levels.

Preparation of the apparatus for both these techniques is of major importance. All apparatus and ampoules of drugs must be autoclaved or gas-sterilised. Drug ampoules should be autoclaved only once and then discarded if not used. Where non-disposable equipment is used, the syringes and needles should be washed finally with distilled water, as even minute traces of detergents can damage the spinal cord. Silicone fluids should never be used to lubricate these syringes, and both syringes and needles should be dismantled before being sterilised.

A variety of indicators are available to aid recognition of the extradural space and the currently popular ones should be included in the pack.

For prolonged operations or post-operative pain control a plastic catheter may be left in the extradural space and intermittent injections given through this.

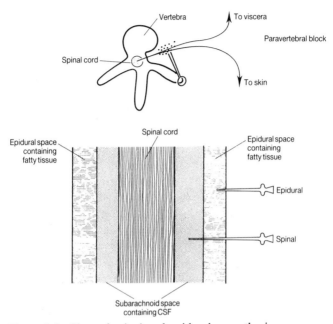

Figure 2.1   Sites of spinal and epidural anaesthesia.

MAINTENANCE OF A GENERAL ANAESTHETIC

Once anaesthetised, the patient must be kept in this condition for the duration of the operation and yet wake as soon as possible afterwards and recover all protective reflexes. Two other conditions are also required during surgery: *analgesia*, to prevent reflex response to pain in light sleep, and *relaxation*, to allow the surgeon access to the abdominal cavity or to allow respiration to be controlled artificially.

Hypnotics keep the patient asleep. Many drugs do this, e.g., intermittent thiopentone, nitrous oxide, and most of the volatile agents.

Analgesia is provided by some anaesthetic gases, volatile agents, or by intravenous opiate alkaloids.

Relaxation may be partial or complete. Muscle relaxants can be used for this purpose.

Muscle relaxants are never given unless some method of ventilating the patient is immediately available.

APPARATUS FOR INHALATION ANAESTHESIA

Boyle's machine

Boyle's machine (Fig. 2.2, p. 48) is the standard British anaesthetic apparatus. Two cylinders of oxygen (black with white shoulders), two of nitrous oxide (blue), and one of carbon dioxide (grey-green) are attached by *pin index* fittings. Each gas has a different *pin index* fitment which will connect only to its own reducing valve. Thus only cylinders of the correct gas can be fitted into the appropriate yokes.

In many operating departments piped gas supplies are available for oxygen and nitrous oxide. The same colour-coding of piped gases applies and the safety precautions to prevent the misconnection of gases hold.

Each gas is passed through a pressure-reducing valve and its own flowmeter; the gases then mix and reach the vaporiser for volatile agents. The mixture then passes into the patient's breathing circuit. The vaporisers vary from the simple screw-top bottle to the Fluotec designed specifically to give accurate known concentrations of volatile agents.

There are four main types of breathing circuits in common use. These are:

1. Magill semi-closed (Fig. 2.3, p. 49)
2. Circle absorber

3. Waters' canister (to-and-fro absorber)
4. Ayre's T-piece (for babies) (Fig. 2.4, p. 49)
   Both (2) and (3) contain soda lime to remove expired carbon dioxide.

Every machine should have in the drawer, on the lower shelf or upper shelf, the following equipment:

- spanner (cylinder key)
- selection of oral airways
- gauze swabs – a different colour from those used by the surgeons in order to avoid confusion in swab counts
- a sphygmomanometer or other more sophisticated electronic equipment to monitor the patient's vital signs
- a mouth gag
- a suction machine should also be available (Fig. 2.5, p. 50 and Fig. 2.6, p. 51)

The rubber parts of the machine are all of antistatic non-conducting rubber to minimise the danger of sparks when using inflammable agents.

ENDOTRACHEAL ANAESTHESIA

Endotracheal intubation assures a patent airway and can provide a gas- and water-tight connection between the patient and the anaesthetic machine (Fig. 2.7, p. 52).

An appropriate size of endotracheal tube (Fig. 2.8, p. 53) is passed through the vocal cords into the trachea with the aid of a laryngoscope. The tube is previously fitted with the largest connector (Fig. 2.9, p. 54) that it will accommodate and the lumen is checked for patency. The catheter mount connects the endotracheal tube to the expiratory valve, and these should be checked for correct fitting and patency.

Indications for endotracheal intubation are:

1. Patients with risk of regurgitation of stomach contents, or blood in the airway.
2. Patients to be artificially ventilated, e.g. those requiring muscle relaxation for thoracic or abdominal surgery.
3. Operations on the head and neck.
4. To remove the anaesthetist from the immediate field of operation.
5. Patients with pre-existing respiratory obstruction.
6. Patients with whom it is difficult to maintain an airway using a mask.
7. Patients lying in prone positions and those with anatomical abnormalities of the face or neck.

Ideally, intubation instruments should be set out on a separate trolley. A wide variety of endotracheal tubes and endotracheal connectors are used, and special tubes are available for endobronchial intubation in chest surgery. Armoured latex tubes are flexible and do not kink but must be stiffened with a wire stilette for introduction. The stilette must never protrude beyond the end of the tube and should be well lubricated to facilitate removal once the tube is in position. Tube sizes are given by internal diameter (ID) in millimetres.

Local anaesthetics may be sprayed over vocal cords and trachea to reduce harmful reflexes. All endotracheal tubes should be sterilised before use.

When uncuffed nasal tubes are used, as in dental or oral surgery, the pharynx is frequently packed off with ribbon gauze. The insertion of such a throat pack should be clearly recorded on the anaesthetic sheet and patient notes.

VENTILATORS

Many machines are now in use which artificially ventilate the patient's lungs (Fig. 2.10, p. 52). This ensures even, regular respiration and releases the anaesthetist's hands to attend to the rest of the patient. All such machines can be switched over to allow the patient to be ventilated manually in the event of mechanical failure.

INTRAVENOUS INFUSIONS AND FLUID THERAPY

There are many different disposable and non-disposable types of needles and cannulae available. These are used for either intermittent or continuous infusions, or continuous injections.

INTRAVENOUS FLUID THERAPY

The total volume of water in the body is expressed as a percentage of body weight, and in adults this ranges from 50 to 70 per cent. Water in the body is distributed among two major compartments: the intracellular fluid (ICF) and the extracellular fluid (ECF).

The ICF comprises approximately two-thirds of the total body water, with the greatest amount residing in the skeletal muscle.

The ECF contains the remaining water, which is divided between the plasma or intravascular fluid compartment and the interstitial fluid compartment.

Although water distribution in the body is described as having specific compartments, it is important to understand that the membranes separating these compartments are freely permeable to water.

The term 'osmosis' refers to the process of water movement across the membrane in response to osmotic pressure. Water always moves from the compartment with the lowest osmotic pressure towards the compartment with the highest osmotic pressure.

Principal ions or electrolytes

ICF	Potassium	K
	Magnesium	Mg
	Phosphates	
	Proteins	

ECF	Sodium	Na
	Chloride	Cl
	Bicarbonate	HCO_3

Because of the abundance of sodium in the ECF, movement of fluids between the ECF and ICF depends chiefly on the concentration of this ion.

Signs of severe water depletion

Apathy or stupor
Lax inelastic skin
Dry mucous membranes

Signs of hypovolaemia

Cold skin
Empty veins
Peripheral cyanosis
Tachycardia
Hypotension
Reduced urinary output, i.e. less than 50 ml/hr.

There are five types of intravenous fluid therapy:

1. Maintenance solutions
2. Replacement solutions
3. Plasma expanders
4. Blood and blood products
5. Total parenteral nutrition.

1. Maintenance solutions

A solution of dextrose 5% in Glucose 5% gives water without electrolytes with little nutritive effect (only 200 k cal/litre). Dextrose is added in order to make the solution isotonic with water.

Sodium chloride 0.18% in 4% dextrose
Sodium chloride 0.3% in 3.3% dextrose.

These two solutions can be used to replace normal losses of water and electrolytes in sweat, expired air, faeces and urine. The normal daily loss of fluid for an adult is 2500 ml/24 hours. This fluid contains 100 m.mol. of sodium and 60 m.mol. of potassium. A common method of maintenance is to give 1 litre of sodium chloride 0.9% plus two litres of 5% Dextrose every 24 hours.

2. Replacement solutions

Hartman's solution, also known as Ringer's solution. This is a compound sodium lactate which contains sodium potassium, calcium chloride and lactate. It is an acceptable substitute to ECF. It is slightly acidic, (pH 6.1). However, once the lactate is metabolised by the liver to bicarbonate, the acidity is buffered. Normal saline (0.9%) is isotonic with plasma and provides a rough approximation to ECF.

Replacement solutions for external losses of intestinal fluids.

NaCl   0.9%
NaCl   0.45%
NaCl   0.9% in 5% dextrose
NaCl   0.9% with 0.3% K.

3. Plasma expanders

Dextrans constitute this group. These are long chains of glucose. Compounds such as Dextran 40 are hypertonic to plasma and therefore increase the plasma volume. Such solutions cause haemodilution, decrease the viscosity of the blood, disaggregate cells, and decrease the adhesiveness of platelets.

Plasma expanders can be used in order to avoid using blood to replace losses of 1 litre or less, or temporarily to maintain circulating volume in more severe haemorrhage.

4. Blood and blood products

These are used to replace the constituent parts of blood or whole blood itself, in those patients who for a variety of reasons have lost blood, or are anaemic.

5. Total parenteral nutrition

This is used to increase the nutritional status of certain patients pre- or post-operatively.

ANAESTHETIC TECHNIQUES AND COMMON DRUGS USED

Total intravenous anaesthesia

This is the technique by which major surgery can be carried out. Respirations are controlled and the lungs are inflated with oxygen-enriched air. Muscle relaxant drugs are used to provide relaxation and therefore prevent reflex muscle movement. The main problem is to assess

Table 2.1

Drug	Dosage	Use
Barbiturates		
Thiopentone	4 mg/Kg	For induction of general anaesthesia
Brietal	1–1.5 mg/Kg	For induction of general anaesthesia
Inhalations		
Halothane	2–5% in O_2	For induction
	0.5–2%	For maintenance of anaesthesia
Nitrous oxide	50–70% in O_2	For maintenance of anaesthesia
Anticholinergics		
Atropine sulphate	300–600 mg	As premedication
	0.6–1.2 mg	For control of neostigmine side-effects
Analgesics		
Papaveretum (Omnopon)	10–20 mg	For premedication 45–60 mins prior to anaesthesia, also during surgery
Muscle relaxants		
Suxemethonium (Scoline) depolarising	20–100 mg	Short duration muscle relaxation used for intubation
Alloferin Competitive blocker	200–250 mcg/Kg	Medium duration muscle relaxant
Anticholinesterases		
Neostigmine methylsulphate (Prostigmin)	1–5 mg with Atropine sulphate 0.6–1.2 mg	Reversal of non-depolarising neuromuscular blockade

Table 2.1 Continued

Drug	Dosage	Use
Antagonists for respiratory depression		
Dopram	1–1.5 mg/Kg	For relieve of post-operative respiratory depression
Narcan	100–200 mcg then adjusted according to response	Reversal of narcotic induced respiratory depression

the depth of anaesthetic given in the paralysed and ventilated patient.

Similar techniques can be used to provide long-term sedation in an Intensive Therapy Unit.

Inhalation anaesthetics

These may be gases or volatile liquids. They can be used both for induction and maintenance of anaesthesia along with intravenous agents.

Gases may be supplied via hospital pipelines or from metal cylinders, all of which are colour-coded. Volatile agents are usually administered using calibrated vaporisers.

To prevent hypoxia, gaseous agents must be given with adequate concentrations of oxygen.

Anticholinergic drugs

These drugs are used to dry the secretions, from bronchi

and salivary glands, which are increased by intubation and anaesthetic gases. They are also used to prevent excessive bradycardia and hypotension.

Sedative and analgesic drugs

Usually given to allay patients' apprehension in the pre-operative period, to relieve pain or discomfort when present and to augment the action of subsequent anaesthetic agents.

Muscle relaxants

Known as 'neuromuscular blocking drugs'. By specific blockade of the neuromuscular junction they enable light levels of anaesthesia to be employed with relaxation of the abdominal muscles and diaphragm. They also relax the vocal cords and allow the passage of an endotracheal tube. Patients who receive a muscle relaxant should *always* have their respiration assisted or controlled until the drug has been inactivated or antagonised.

Depolarising muscle relaxants

These drugs act by mimicking the action of Acetylcholine at the neuromuscular junction and cause blockade. Depolarisation is prolonged since their break-away from the receptor site and subsequent breakdown are slower than for Acetylcholine. This provides short-term muscle relaxation.

Non-depolarising muscle relaxants

These are also known as competitive blockers. They cause blockade by competing with Acetylcholine at the receptor site and neuromuscular junction. They are best suited to the production of paralysis of a long duration.

Their action, unlike depolarising muscle relaxants, can be reversed with Anticholinesterases.

Anticholinesterases

These drugs reverse the action of competitive blockers, but they prolong the action of depolarising drugs. They cause muscarinic reactions, especially excessive salivation and bradycardia.

SOME COMPLICATIONS OF ANAESTHESIA

Respiratory obstruction

This is a very common complication which is potentially hazardous. It can lead to coughing, straining and regurgitation, and can result in hypoxaemia and a reduction in the depth of anaesthesia. The most common causes of respiratory obstruction during anaesthesia are the following:

- The patient's lips being tightly closed together.
- The tongue falling back into the oropharynx.
- Some form of mechanical obstruction – e.g., the catheter mount may twist and obstruct, or the endotracheal tube may kink.
- The endotracheal tube may have been over-inflated, causing herniation of the cuff over the distal end of the tube.
- The distal orifice of the endotracheal tube may be lying against the wall of the trachea.
- The endotracheal tube may be too long for the patient and endobronchial intubation has actually taken place.

Respiratory obstruction can be recognised in the anaesthetised patient by snoring, inadequate movement of the reservoir bag, or an obstructed respiratory pattern.

If the cause is mechanical, then correction of the fault will clear the obstruction.

Bronchospasm

This complication can arise when:

- The endotracheal tube is too near the bronchial carina.
- The anaesthetic is too light for the surgical stimulation taking place.
- The patient aspirates some stomach contents.

This complication can be recognised by the presence of an audible wheeze, a prolonged expiratory phase and if an increased inflation pressure is required.

If bronchospasm occurs, it is important to maintain and achieve adequate oxygenation while treating the spasm with an intravenous injection or infusion of either Aminophylline 250 mg or Salbutamol 25 mg.

Laryngeal spasm

This complication can occur:

- During induction of anaesthesia.
- Due to the premature insertion of an artificial airway or laryngoscope.
- Due to the presence of pharyngeal secretions, or vomit.
- At the stage of surgical incision when anaesthesia is too light.
- During specific surgical interventions; e.g. anal stretch, breast surgery and dilation of cervix.
- Following extubation.

Laryngeal spasm can be recognised by a growing inspiratory noise which may progress to complete spasm. This will lead to hypoxaemia. It can be treated with 100 per cent oxygen given with respiratory assistance. If the patient requires to be intubated, then Suxamethonium is given intravenously to allow endotracheal intubation of the larynx. If the spasm occurs following endotracheal extubation, then Doxapram is given.

Hiccoughs

This complication can occur as a result of vagal stimulation by specific anaesthetic agents. It is usually prevented by the use of Hyoscine or Atropine for premedication.

Hypotension

This is defined when systolic arterial pressure falls below 90 mmHg and can occur as a result of:

- Hypovolaemia.
- The administration of certain anaesthetic induction agents such as Halothane, Enflurane or Isoflurane.
- The administration of certain muscle relaxants, e.g. Tubocurarine.
- Cardiovascular disease.
- Respiratory disease or pneumothorax.
- Hypersensitivity reactions.

Generally this is treated with intravenous fluids and/or Ephedrine.

Hypertension

This can occur when:

- The anaesthesia is too light.
- There is inadequate analgesia.
- There is inadequate hypnosis.
- The patient starts to cough or strain on the endotracheal tube.

- The patient has existing hypertension.
- The aorta is cross-clamped during vascular surgery.
- The patient is hypercapnic.
- Certain drugs have been used; e.g. Adrenaline, Ergometrine or Ketamine.

Halothane may be used to control hypertension.

Malignant hyperpyrexia

This is a potentially fatal, inherited abnormality in skeletal muscle cells. Individuals who have this predisposition may, when exposed to certain anaesthetic agents, experience a rapid increase in body temperature of at least 2°C per hour.

Halothane and Suxamethonium are the two drugs most likely to produce the condition, although all volatile anaesthetic agents should be avoided in an individual who is known to be susceptible. Lignocaine should also be avoided.

Malignant hyperpyrexia can be recognised by:

- An increased muscle tone following injection of Suxamethonium.
- Hyperpyrexia appears later during anaesthesia or in the early post-operative period.
- Tachycardia.
- Hyperpnoea.
- Cyanosis.
- Hypoxaemia.
- Metabolic acidosis.
- Hyperkalaemia (abnormal high potassium level in blood).
- Hypercalcaemia (excess of calcium in blood).
- Tetany (sharp flexion of wrist and ankle joints, muscle twitchings, cramps, convulsion attacks of stridor).
- Myoglobinuria (presence of oxygen-carrying pigment of muscle in urine).
- Acute renal failure.
- Cardiac failure.

The treatment for malignant hyperpyrexia during anaesthesia is to discontinue the volatile anaesthetic agent being used, administer 100 per cent oxygen, swathe the patient in ice or ice packs, and administer sodium bicarbonate to treat acidosis and insulin to treat hyperkalaemia. The drug available for the specific treatment of malignant hyperpyrexia is Dantrolene. This should be given intravenously and repeated every 5–10 mins up to the maximum dose until control of the condition has been obtained.

Regurgitation of stomach contents

This complication is seldom accompanied by an outward sign or sound from the patient, and occurs when the patient is in a deeper level of unconsciousness, by which time the cough reflexes are either less active than normal or totally absent. Unless adequate precautions have been taken inhalation of the gastric contents will certainly occur.

Regurgitation of stomach contents can occur when:

- The patient's stomach has not been emptied prior to surgery.
- The patient vomits during the pre-operative period.
- The patient has a specific illness which causes delayed gastric emptying.
- Specific anaesthetic agents are administered.
- The patient receives topical anaesthetic to vocal cords.

Where there is a risk of regurgitation, the preventive measure of applying cricoid pressure is best. If regurgitation has taken place, the patient's head should be lowered and the mouth cleared using suction apparatus.

Table 2.2

Name	Actions
Alcuronium	Medium long-acting muscle relaxant which may cause histamine release, hypotension, tachycardia; commonly used non-depolarising relaxant.
Alfentanil	A short-acting synthetic opiate used intravenously during anaesthesia to provide intense analgesia and sedation.
Atracurium	A short- to medium-acting non-depolarising muscle relaxant which undergoes spontaneous hydrolysis in the body to an inactive product. It may cause histamine release and bradycardia. Because of its self-destructive hydrolysis, it is most useful in patients with renal disease as it does not require renal excretion.
Atropine	An anticholinergic. It is used in three situations in anaesthesia: (1) premedication, to dry secretions and to protect the heart by partially blocking the vagus nerve; (2) during anaesthesia to speed the heart where bradycardia has occurred; (3) at the end of anaesthesia to block the side-effects of the anticholinesterase given to reverse neuromuscular blockade.
Bubivacaine	A long-acting local anaesthetic, used for local anaesthesia where the duration of block is important.
Carbon dioxide	A gas which may be used to stimulate respiration during gaseous induction or at the termination of IPPV (Intermittent Positive Pressure Ventilation).
Curare	Generic name for non-depolarising muscle relaxants most frequently used are Alcuronium, Pancuronium, Atracurium, Vecuronium and Tubocurarine.

Table 2.2 Continued

Name	Actions
Doxapram	Respiratory stimulant – causes patient to hyperventilate, also causes central arousal.
Droperidol	Major tranquilliser which causes catatonia and can be used in combination with intravenous opiate to produce 'Neuroleptanalgesia' – and with opiate plus nitrous oxide, 'Neuroleptanaesthesia'. Very potent anti-emetic.
Enflurane	Anaesthetic vapour of the substituted ether group. Potent anaesthetic and analgesic; also potent respiratory and circulatory depressant.
Ether	The original anaesthetic vapour. Potent anaesthetic and analgesic but inflammable and explosive – maintains respiration and circulation until very deep anaesthesia, unlike other vapours currently available – very slow uptake and induction if sole agent used. Rarely used nowadays.
Etomidate	Intravenous induction agent, causing rapid loss of consciousness but not complete loss of reflex activity. Can also be used as infusion (along with an opiate) to produce total intra-venous anaesthesia.
Fentanyl	Short-acting, very potent opiate analgesic producing profound sedation, analgesia and respiratory depression.
Glycopyrrolate	Atropine-like agent, used for same indications – longer-acting than atropine.

Table 2.2 Continued

Name	Actions
Halothane	Commonly used anaesthetic vapour. Potent anaesthetic with little analgesic activity. Rapid in uptake and can be used for rapid gaseous induction – non-irritant in comparison with other anaesthetic vapours. Causes increasing respiratory depression in line with increasing depth of anaesthesia. Causes slowing of heart and hypotension both by cardiac and vascular activity. Associated with occasional cases of jaundice post-operatively.
Hyoscine	Atropine-like drug – which crosses into the brain to cause good sedation in adults. May cause excitation in children and the elderly. Also potent antiemetic.
Isoflurane	Anaesthetic vapour – substituted ether group – potent anaesthetic and analgesic but too pungent to be used for gaseous induction. Causes more respiratory depression than Halothane but less than Enflurane. Does not cause cardiac depression but drops the blood pressure by direct vascular ability. May be rarely associated with post-operative jaundice.
Ketamine	An intravenous induction and maintenance agent causing dissociative anaesthesia – very potent analgesic. Dissociative anaesthesia is unlike normal anaesthesia in that the patient may appear awake, look around, move, even vocalise, but is insensible to pain or stimuli. Causes rise in blood pressure, tachycardia and bronchodilation; the last makes it useful in asthmatics.

Table 2.2 Continued

Name	Actions
Lignocaine	The standard local anaesthetic solution. Causes local numbness and motor weakness on injection. Side-effects include arrythmias and convulsions, but these are due to overdose. Comes in solution with or without Adrenaline.
Methadone	A long-acting opiate used as an alternative to Papaveretum, Pethidine, etc., for pre-medication and post-operative analgesia but is rarely used intra-operatively.
Methohexitone	An intravenous induction agent of the Barbiturate group. May cause convulsions during induction in susceptible patients. Induces unconsciousness rapidly. Less irritant to veins than Thiopentone but causes pain on injection. More rapidly metabolised post-operatively than Thiopentone.
Metoclopramide	Antiemetic – used post-operatively to reduce nausea and vomiting associated with anaesthesia and opiates. Can be used pre-operatively to hasten gastric emptying in emergency.
Nalbuphine	Minor opiate which can be used to produce analgesia or sedation when given alone – or to reverse effect of more potent opiate given previously.
Naloxone	An opiate antagonist. It reverses the analgesic and respiratory depressant effects of Morphine, Methadone, Fentanyl, Pethidine, Papaveretum, etc. Has no analgesic or respiratory effects of its own.

Table 2.2 Continued

Name	Actions
Neostigmine	Anticholinesterase which can be used to reverse the action of non-depolarising muscle relaxants at the end of operation but also acts on the autonomic nervous system – increasing the secretions, slowing heart, causing spasm in the bowel, so Atropine is given along with it to block these side-effects.
Nitrous oxide	Anaesthetic gas. Very weak anaesthetic – very difficult to use as sole anaesthetic but in combination with a vapour very good, as it is a potent analgesic.
Oxygen	Gas used as basic carrier for anaesthetic vapours. Essential for life, oxygen is used in place of air as anaesthesia alters lung dynamics requiring a high inspired concentration of oxygen to maintain levels in the blood. Also vapour and gases would dilute the oxygen in air, rendering the mixture hypoxic.
Pancuronium	Non-depolarising muscle relaxant – long-acting. Does not cause histamine release – causes hypertension and tachycardia.
Papaveretum	Standardised mixture of opium alkaloids. Overall effect is to produce analgesia with less vomiting than with morphine alone.
Pentazocine	Minor opiate which on its own produces analgesia and sedation – but if given following major opiate, reverses that drug's effects.
Perphenazine	Potent antiemetic and sedative used in pre-medication to increase sedation or drowsiness and act as antiemetic. Used post-operatively also to reduce emetic side-effects of opiates.

Table 2.2 Continued

Name	Actions
Pethidine	Synthetic opiate. Used in premedication, intra-operatively to deepen anaesthesia, and post-operatively for analgesia. Unlike most opiates, does not cause spasm of smooth muscle and is therefore useful in various colics (renal, biliary) and in asthma.
Phenoperidine	Synthetic opiate – more potent than Pethidine but causes more respiratory depression.
Prochlorperazine	Antiemetic and sedative of the major tranquilliser group. Used for sedation and post-operatively to reduce vomiting.
Propofol	Anaesthetic induction agent with minor side-effects.
Pyridostigmine	Long-acting anticholinesterase used to reverse the action of non-depolarising muscle relaxants. Has less action on the autonomic nervous system than Neostigmine.
Suxamethonium	Depolarising muscle relaxant – acts in a different way from other muscle relaxants, produces rapid, profound muscle relaxation. Suitable for intubation. Causes patients to fasciculate (fine muscle twitching) as they become paralysed. Cannot be reversed – must be allowed to wear off spontaneously.
Thiopentone	Intravenous induction agent of the barbiturate group. Induces unconsciousness rapidly. Very irritant to blood vessels, causing thrombophlebitis, but painless on injection into veins. Very slowly metabolised/excreted post-operatively, although recovery of consciousness from a single dose is rapid.

Table 2.2 Continued

Name	Actions
Tubocurarine	The original non-depolarising muscle relaxant – extracted from South American arrow poisons. Long-acting. Causes histamine release, hypotension and bradycardia due to ganglion blocking effects. Stable in solution.
Vecuronium	Non-depolarising muscle relaxant of medium duration. Rapidly metabolised in the liver. Does not cause histamine release; does not have any cardiovascular effects.

Source: Developed from a teaching handout produced by Dr John G. Muir (1986), Aberdeen Royal Infirmary.

PAEDIATRIC ANAESTHESIA

This section has been included so as to provide an insight into the key differences between neonates and adults in terms of physiology and anaesthetic requirements. The most obvious difference is size and the body mass index of the neonate and the adult. There are key anatomical and physiological differences also.

General metabolism

At rest, the oxygen requirement of the average adult is approximately 3 ml/kg/min. From the first week of life the resting oxygen consumption of a neonate is approximately 9 ml/kg/min. Such a high oxygen requirement has the following implications for anaesthesia:

1. During respiration, oxygen is converted into carbon dioxide. In a neonate the output of this gas is three times that of an adult. In order to excrete such an amount of carbon dioxide, the pulmonary ventilation

of a neonate is about 3 times that of an adult. To achieve this the neonate respiratory rate is increased. Therefore, during anaesthesia the type of apparatus used and the amount of ventilation required must enable the child to eliminate carbon dioxide effectively.

2. If respiratory obstruction or cardiac arrest occurs during anaesthesia, the oxygen supplies are used up 3 times more quickly than in the adult. Consequently, a neonate will experience hypoxaemia much more quickly than an adult.

3. As water and energy turnover are directly related to oxygen consumption, children are much more susceptible to dehydration and hypoglycaemia during anaesthesia.

4. Neonates have a high resting cardiac output (3 times that of adults) in order to supply sufficient oxygen and carbohydrates to the body cells and to remove waste products.

Respiratory system

The main anatomical differences between adults and children occur in the upper airway. In the child the tongue is larger, the lower jaw smaller, the epiglottis is floppy and folds on itself. All these differences may effect endotracheal intubation.

The narrowest part of a child's airway (until age 8–10) is the cricoid cartilage. If the correct size of endotracheal tube is chosen there will be an airtight fit without inflating the cuff. It is further important not to use too tight an endotracheal tube as this may cause oedematous swelling of the cricoid mucosa post-operatively. This can result in an upper respiratory obstruction. The best fit is one which produces a slight leak when positive pressure is applied to the airway. In children under 10 the cricoid cartilage is narrower than the nasal tubes, so an airtight fit can be achieved with both oral and nasal tubes.

Sometimes, following intubation, an oropharyngeal pack is used. This helps stabilise the tube and soak up secretions. As with adults, the length of the tube is important. An endotracheal tube cut too short can become displaced from the trachea, and a tube which is too long will enter the right main bronchus.

Intubation

In the neonate, intubation is usually carried out whilst the baby is awake, for safety reasons. For, once a baby is anaesthetised and paralysed, trouble may be experienced in ventilating the baby using a mask. Cyanosis frequently occurs during awake intubation due to coughing and breath-holding. A suction catheter passed through the nose into the pharynx and oxygen administered help to prevent cyanosis.

Pulmonary ventilation

In neonates, as in adults, the diaphragm plays an important role in ventilation. In the child, however, the thoracic component is much reduced due to the ribs being almost horizontal and cartilagenous.

In the event of respiratory obstruction, the ribs are sucked inwards by the action of the diaphragm and therefore tend to decrease lung expansion. This makes the diaphragm less efficient. With neonates, low-resistance, wide-bore anaesthetic apparatus should be used. Neonatal anaesthetic equipment should have a low resistance and also a low dead space.

The tidal volume of the average neonate is approximately 20 ml, of which 6–8 ml is classified as 'dead space'. This means that only 12–14 ml of inspired gases actually take part in alveolar ventilation.

Anaesthetic circuits

Rendell-Baker apparatus: This consists of a wide-bore plate. Fresh gas flows on one side of the plate, and passes over the child's face up the other side of the plate and out through a piece of wide-bore tubing into a bag with a hole in the bottom. The child, therefore, inhales from a constant stream of fresh gas and there is limited dead space.

The Ayre's T piece is mainly used during endotracheal anaesthesia. It is small and can easily be fixed to a child's face. Fresh gas is provided by a side arm and on expiration passes down the wide-bore tubing to a bag with a hole in the bottom and out to the atmosphere or to a scavenging system. The bag allows artificial ventilation to be used, by closing the end and squeezing. These two circuits are best suited for the ages newborn to 3 years.

Humidification and warming of gases

This may be done to prevent heat loss by inhalation of dry gases at room temperature. Furthermore, dry gases have a detrimental effect upon tracheal and bronchial mucosa in children.

Heat loss and temperature control

Babies in the age bracket 3–6 months are unable to control body temperature effectively. During surgery there are many sources of heat loss. For example:

- A child has a greater surface area, weight for weight, than an adult, therefore heat loss to the atmosphere is greater.
- Anaesthesia produces vasodilation, therefore heat is lost from the skin.
- In some neonates there is very little fat and therefore very little natural insulation.

- Heat can be lost from evaporation from surgical wounds, or infusion of cold intravenous fluids.
- Neonates cannot shiver and therefore cannot create heat.

The following measures may be taken to avoid heat loss during surgery:

1. Raise theatre temperature.
2. Place the child on a warm mattress, covered with gauze to prevent burns.
3. Cover the child with gauze, apart from operating site.
4. Cover child with a 'space blanket'.
5. Warm all intravenous fluids.
6. Warm the anaesthetic gases.

However, if the child is over 6 months of age, these precautions may be reduced to prevent hyperthermia.

Care of the child during induction of anaesthesia requires great skill in order to relieve anxiety and to ensure a safe intubation. The nurse working in this speciality must be aware of the normal range of vital signs for a child, and paediatric drug dosages. In addition, recent research has indicated that parental or significant other presence in the anaesthetic room reduces the child's fear; where appropriate, the theatre nurse and anaesthetist may encourage this.

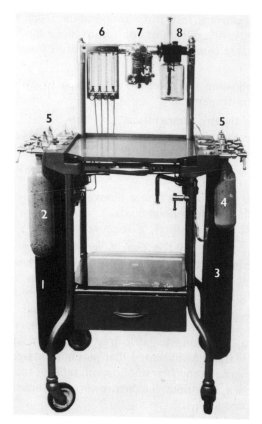

Figure 2.2 Boyle's machine.
1. Oxygen cylinders
2. Carbon dioxide cylinder
3. Nitrous oxide cylinders
4. Cyclopropane cylinder
5. Pin index connections
6. Flowmeters
7. Fluotec vaporiser
8. Bottle vaporiser (rarely used nowadays)

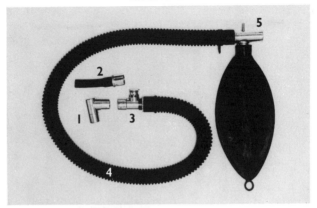

Figure 2.3 Magill semi-closed circuit.
1. Angled mask mount
2. Endotracheal catheter mount
3. Expiratory valve
4. Corrugated tube
5. Machine-to-bag mount

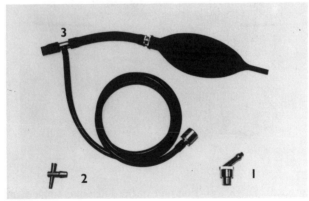

Figure 2.4 Ayre's T-piece (Jackson-Rees modification)
(used for neonates and infants up to 15 kg).
1. Universal mask mount
2. Cardiff endotracheal tube mount
3. Ayre's T-piece connector

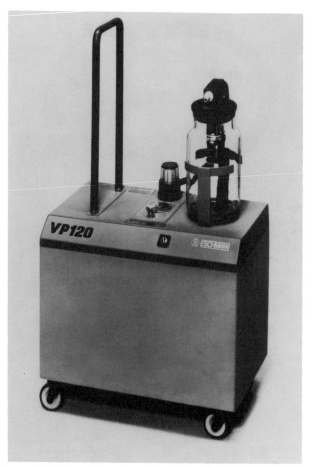

Figure 2.5 Surgical suction unit of the single-jar, single-pump type.

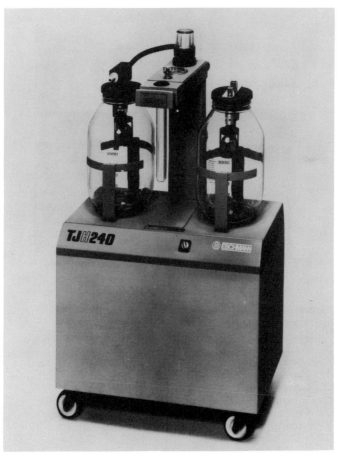

Figure 2.6 Twin suction unit for use in anaesthetic room.

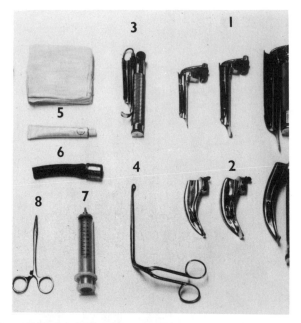

Figure 2.7 Intubation instruments.
1. Magill laryngoscope (straight blade) three sizes
2. Macintosh laryngoscope (curved blade) three sizes
3. Anderson infant laryngoscope
4. Magill intubating forceps
5. Coloured gauze swabs and lubricant. (*N.B.* lubricant from tube – never from communal multi-used jar)
6. Endotracheal catheter mount
7. Cuff inflating syringe
8. Spencer-Wells haemostat to clip inflated cuffed tube

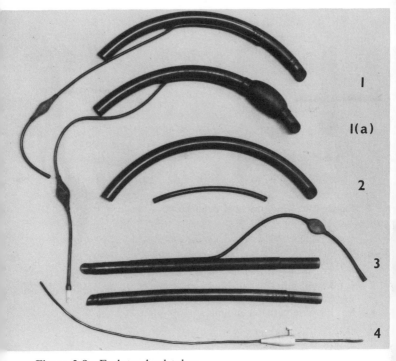

Figure 2.8 Endotracheal tubes.
1.   Cuffed oral Magill tube
1(a) Same with cuff inflated
2.   Uncuffed tubes, showing size range (3 mm–12 mm internal diameter)
3.   Armoured latex tubes, cuffed and plain
4.   Introducing stilette for armoured tubes

The tubes shown are latex endotracheal tubes which are non-disposable. In many operating departments disposable tubes are in use.

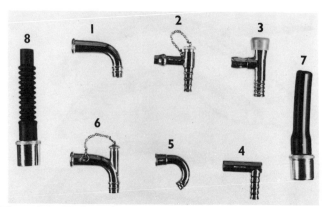

Figure 2.9   Endotracheal connectors.
1.   Magill universal
2.   Cobbs suction
3.   Magill suction
4.   Rowbotham
5.   Magill nasal
6.   Magill universal suction
7.   Straight catheter mount
8.   Flexible catheter mount

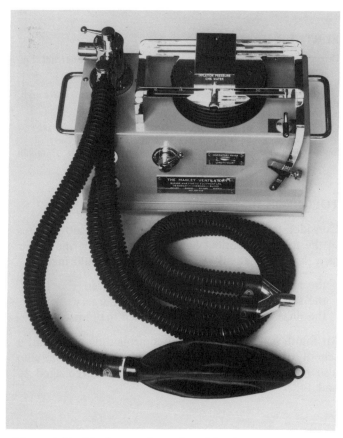

Figure 2.10 Manley ventilator (gas-driven).

FURTHER READING

Brigden, R.J. (1990) *Operating Theatre Technique*, Churchill Livingstone, Edinburgh.

Campbell, D. and Spence, A. (1980) *A Nurse's Guide to Anaesthetics, Resuscitation and Intensive Care*, Churchill Livingstone, Edinburgh.

Carrie, L.E.S. and Simpson, P.J. (1982) *Understanding Anaesthesia*, Heinemann, London.

Ostlere, G. and Bryce-Smith, R. (1980) *Anaesthetics for Medical Students*, Churchill Livingstone, Edinburgh.

Smith, G. and Aikenhead A.R. (eds) (1989) *Anaesthesia*, Churchill Livingstone, Edinburgh.

TOPIC FOR DISCUSSION: ANAESTHESIA

Consider the anaesthetic advantages and disadvantages of the following patient having an inguinal hernia repair as a day case patient. Your discussions should include:

the anaesthetic drugs which could be used
the suitability of the patient for day surgery
the anaesthetic complications which may arise

Mr Smith is 44 years old, diet-controlled diabetic, and a school-teacher. He lives in a large city with his wife who also teaches full-time. They have two children aged 16 and 14.

3   Intra-operative patient care

This chapter will focus on various aspects of patient care during a surgical procedure. In the operating department the nurse can expect to participate as a member of the surgical team, either in the circulating or scrub nurse role.

Whilst involved in intra-operative patient care in the operating department the nurse can expect to:

- participate in the planning of operating sessions and the management of an operating list.
- assess, plan and implement the total care of the unconscious or sedated patient.
- coordinate and document planned patient care during the intra-operative phase.
- create a safe and therapeutic environment for both patients and staff.
- practise the correct wearing of theatre apparel.
- always practise according to the principles of asepsis.
- communicate effectively with other members of the surgical team.

THE ROLE AND RESPONSIBILITIES OF THE SCRUBBED ASSISTANT

The scrubbed assistant is the member of staff who prepares the sterilised instruments and equipment ready for the operation: this may be a nurse or an operating department assistant.

Before the operation the scrubbed assistant's duties are to

1. Check the surgeon's preference card and collect the specialised equipment, sutures and instrument and bowl sets.
2. Gown and glove, using an aseptic technique.
3. (a) Drape the trolleys and bowl stands with sterile drapes, if pre-packed sets are not in use, *or* (b) Drape the trolleys and bowl stands with the sterile drapes contained within the pre-packed instrument trays.
4. Check the contents of each instrument set with the circulator and with the enclosed content list.
5. Collect from the circulator sutures, needles, blades and other necessary sterile equipment.
6. Check swabs, packs, instruments and needles with the circulator in accordance with local procedure and the recommendations of the Medical Defence Union and the Royal College of Nursing and the National Association of Theatre Nurses.
7. Ensure that the findings are charted and displayed.
8. Drape additional tables, trolleys as required.
9. Request the circulator to check the patient's identity with name band, case notes and operating list.
10. When the patient arrives in the theatre, ensure that he or she is positioned safely on the operating table.

At the commencement of the operation, the scrubbed assistant:

11. Hands the skin preparation and sponges on a sponge-holder to the surgeon.
12. Assists in applying and securing drapes.
13. Positions the trolleys and bowl stands.
14. Hands the diathermy leads and suction tubing

to the circulator for attachment and checks the diathermy setting with the surgeon.

15. Prepares on a working surface the following items:
    scalpel
    dissecting scissors
    small artery forceps
    toothed and non-toothed dissecting forceps
    diathermy equipment

16. Hands swabs to the surgeon and assistant surgeon.

17. Passes instruments, swabs and sutures as needed, replacing instruments on the working surface with others from the trolley as the operation proceeds.

18. Keeps an accurate count of extra swabs, needles or instruments collected during the operation and ensures that they are charted by the circulator.

19. Anticipates the needs of the surgeon by continually observing the progress of the operation.

20. Ensures that noise and movement within the theatre is kept to a minimum.

Before the surgeon sutures any cavity, the scrubbed assistant:

21. Checks swabs, packs, instruments and needles with the circulator in accordance with local procedure, informs the surgeon of the findings, and ensures that the surgeon acknowledges the information.

At the end of the operation, the scrubbed assistant:

22. Checks with the circulator that the appropriate wound dressing is available.

23. Carries out a final check, informs the surgeon, and ensures that the findings are charted.

24. Removes instruments from the working surface.

25. Collects the dressing from the circulator for the surgeon.
26. Removes blades from scalpel handles and disposes of used blades, needles, and other sharps in the appropriate container.
27. Removes the drapes from the patient.
28. Ensures that the area around the wound dressing is clean and that the patient's gown and sheet are clean and dry.
29. Covers the patient with a clean sheet.
30. Degowns and degloves.

When the anaesthetist gives permission, the scrubbed assistant accompanies the patient to the recovery room and gives all relevant information to the recovery nurse.

On returning to the theatre, the scrubbed assistant completes the entry in the register and signs it, checks the instrument set and other equipment, and either returns them to the TSSU (theatre surgical supplies unit) or washes them and prepares them for sterilisation, as appropriate.

THE ROLE AND RESPONSIBILITIES OF THE CIRCULATOR

The term 'circulator' is used in many hospitals to refer to the 'runner', i.e. the nurse or operating department assistant who helps the scrubbed assistant to prepare for the operation and is available throughout the procedure.

Before the operation, the circulator:

1. Checks that the theatre has been cleaned and that the suction apparatus, diathermy equipment and the operating lights are in working order.
2. Ensures that the temperature and humidity controls are correctly set.
3. Collects the necessary stock and equipment, e.g.

swabs, specimen jar, sterile water, fibre-optic light source.

4. Prepares sterilised gowns and gloves for the team and assists in tying gowns.
5. Opens instrument and bowl-packs and other necessary equipment for the scrubbed assistant.
6. Assists with the count and records the count on a display board.

During the operation, the circulator:

7. Remains in the theatre throughout.
8. Connects the diathermy and suction leads to the appropriate machinery.
9. Replenishes and records swabs and packs as requested.
10. Adheres strictly to local policy for disposal of used swabs.
11. Fills bowls with sterile water, if required.
12. Ensures that all theatre doors remain closed.
13. Places swab-collecting bowls conveniently for the scrubbed assistant and surgical team.
14. Anticipates the requirements of the surgical team.
15. Records the blood loss as appropriate.

Before the end of the operation, the circulator:

16. Assists with the count and records.
17. Prepares the wound dressing.

On completion of the operation, the circulator:

18. Hands the dressing to the scrubbed assistant.
19. Helps with the removal of drapes and the preparation of the patient for return to the recovery room.
20. Removes the instrument trolley and other equipment to the dirty utility area.
21. Ensures that the theatre is cleaned and prepared for the next case.

Figures 3.1–3.5 show the sequence of preparation of the sterile trolley.

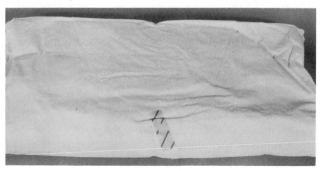

Figure 3.1 The circulator or runner places the sterilised pack on the trolley and removes the outer cover.

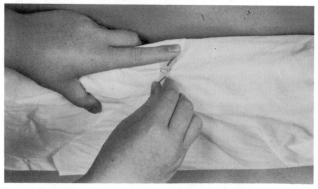

Figure 3.2 The inner pack is carefully opened.

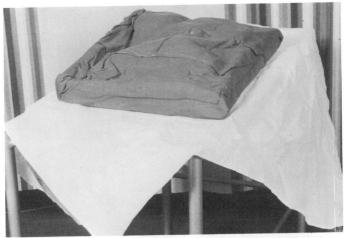

Figure 3.3 The paper wrap is carefully draped over the trolley by the circulator, who touches the outside of the paper only.

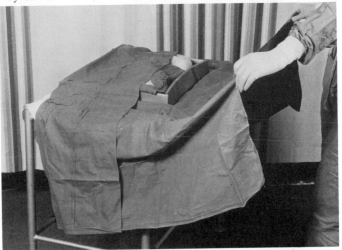

Figure 3.4 The scrubbed person picks up the sterile drape.

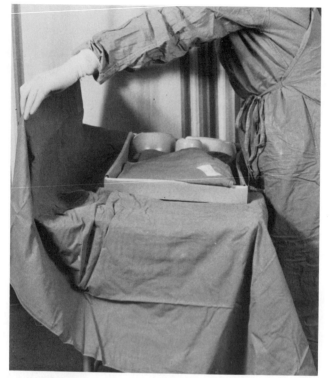

Figure 3.5 The sterile drape is used to drape the trolley.

POSITIONING THE PATIENT

Once anaesthesia has been established, the patient is positioned for surgery. The patient's notes and operating list are again checked to identify the correct site, and the surgeon will check the position before commencing the operation. The nurse removes the patient's gown, if necessary, but ensures that he is not unnecessarily exposed. The unconscious patient is totally dependent on the staff who are caring for him, and the nurse, as the patient's advocate, should ensure that he is treated with dignity and respect.

Pressure points are protected and the appropriate supports for the operation are positioned. Particular care should be taken with the old and infirm, and information collected during the pre-operative visit should ensure that any deformity or physical handicap is known to the theatre nursing staff. If diathermy is to be used during the operation, the diathermy pad will be applied at this stage. At the end of the operation, all pressure points should be checked to ensure that no damage has been caused to the patient.

Prevention of complications

As the patient will be positioned on the operating table and may remain so for several hours it is necessary that the nurse ensures that the patient receives the best possible care and that where possible complications are pre-empted. This requires that the nurse plans care in advance and is knowledgeable of the needs of the patient.

In many operating departments the positioning of patients for surgery is carried out by medical and nursing staff following anaesthesia. Positioning is potentially dangerous for the patient unless the utmost care is taken. The aims of positioning patients for surgery are as follows:

- to maintain anatomical alignment.
- to provide support where appropriate.
- to ensure that the patient is stable and secure on the operating table.
- to prevent injuries to the skin and prominences.
- to provide exposure of the operating site.

Musculo-skeletal problems

These problems can occur when a patient is positioned incorrectly. Certain elderly or infirm patients may be unable to be positioned in the ideal way. If these problems are not recognised prior to anaesthesia, then it is possible to damage the patient.

The raising or lowering of limbs in unison for certain positions prevents damage. Nerves can also be damaged when either compressed or stretched by the hyperextension of a joint. Care is needed to ensure that the arms of patients are not hyperextended. Generally, during major surgery, one of the patient's arms will be extended on an arm-board, which is then abducted. When this occurs it is essential, in order to prevent damage to the brachial plexus, that the angle of abduction does not exceed 90 degrees.

Skin problems

As with the lifting of any patient, it is necessary to follow good kinetic lifting principles so as to avoid personal back injury and friction or shearing damage to the patient. Within the operating department, many aids are available to assist with the lifting of patients. These vary from lateral transfer trolleys and operating tables, to rollers, or slides, to transfer patients on to beds. In situations where an aid is either not appropriate or available, then a three-person lift will be used to transfer the anaesthetised patient.

Skin and soft tissue can easily be damaged by pressure and, where appropriate, padding can be used to minimise the risk.

Ocular problems

Damage to the patient's eyes can occur from secretions, from intra-ocular pressure or from corneal abrasions.

Circulatory problems

During a general anaesthetic, a patient's blood pressure may be altered. In addition during long periods of immobility, and venous stagnation can occur. It is therefore necessary that precautions are taken to minimise these possibilities. The use of thrombo-embolitic deterrent stockings or alternating pressure leggings assist with venous return and are of value to patients undergoing major surgery.

Alternatively, raising the lower limbs slightly helps to prevent pressure and assist with blood flow. This will be suitable for certain patients.

Equipment used during positioning

The operating table is a complex and sophisticated piece of equipment which requires to be mastered. Tables can have mechanical or electronic controls. All operating tables are articulated in order to position patients. They can be locked in position and are also mobile. Each table can accommodate securely a range of attachments and extensions. The mattress of the table is usually 2 inches thick and is covered with smooth antistatic bonded rubber. (Figures 3.6 to 3.20 at the end of the chapter illustrate the operating table, various surgical positions and table attachments).

During surgery, water mattresses, alternating pressure mattresses, or vacuum pack mattresses may be used in addition to assist with the care of particular patients. These mattresses are easily accommodated on top of the rubber operating table mattress.

PATIENT CARE DURING ELECTRO-SURGERY

'Diathermy' is the term used in surgery to control haemorrhage or to cut through tissue. There are two types of
diathermy: *monopolar* and *bipolar*. To enable the specialist
equipment (Fig. 3.21, p. 82) to be used competently, it is
essential that the nurse understands the electro-physics and
mechanics of the equipment whilst it is in use.

Monopolar diathermy

In monopolar diathermy a high-frequency current is
passed through the patient's body from the live electrode
to the indifferent electrode. The live electrode is the
specially insulated surgeon's diathermy 'forceps or pencil'.
The indifferent electrode is the 'diathermy pad' attached
to the patient and the diathermy machine.

When the surgeon uses the diathermy forceps or pencil,
the narrow entry point of the current results in high tissue
resistance, which in turn creates a very local high
temperature. This high temperature is used to control
haemorrhage by coagulation or to cut tissues by cell
disruption. The current then continues to the indifferent
electrode and hence to earth.

If the current is diverted from the comparatively large
area of the indifferent electrode and finds an alternative
path from the patient to earth, tissue damage may occur
due to the high resistance at the point of exit. The most
likely alternative pathway is created by the patient coming
into contact with a metal part of the operating table.

Bipolar diathermy

In bipolar diathermy the live and indifferent electrodes
are combined within the handle of the diathermy forceps.
These electrodes are separated by insulating material.

When in use, the current passes from one electrode to the other at the point of contact. There is no need to use a patient diathermy pad (indifferent electrode) when using bipolar diathermy as the circuit is completed between the points of the forceps. Bipolar diathermy can be used for coagulation only and is therefore restricted in applicability. As with any electrical equipment, safety precautions are necessary.

Safety precautions

In most operating departments monopolar diathermy is most widely used. Before using any diathermy equipment, whether monopolar or bipolar, special safety checks must be carried out to ensure that the equipment is in good working order and to prevent injury to either the patient or the operator. The use of antistatic material on table mattresses, pillows and theatre staff footwear is essential.

The insulation on all cables and equipment must be intact and the recommended procedures for checking the alarm systems followed. Diathermy machines generally have integral alarm systems which sound when there is any disruption or untoward alteration in the circuit. The live electrode is usually controlled by a foot-switch or switch on the handle of the forceps which connects to the diathermy machine.

During surgery, the live electrode or diathermy forceps are usually kept in an insulated container (diathermy quiver) away from the operative field. The members of the surgical team must take care to avoid standing on the foot-switch when the diathermy forceps are not in use.

Application of the indifferent electrode (diathermy pad)

The indifferent electrode is most effective when applied over a vascular and muscular area of the patient's body, such as under the thigh, or the buttock. To ensure good conduction, the diathermy pad (indifferent electrode) must be:

- In direct and complete contact with the patient.
- Dry.
- As close to the operative site as is practical.
- Secured to the patient before connection to the diathermy machine in order to avoid potential burns.

Prior to applying and on removal of the diathermy pad, the condition of the patient's skin at and around the site of the pad should be checked for any damage or injury.

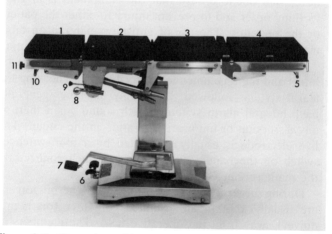

Figure 3.6 Operating table with radiolucent top.
1.   Detachable head section
     (interchangeable with leg section)
2.   Upper trunk section
3.   Lower trunk section

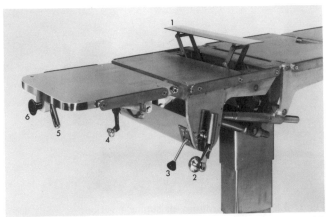

Figure 3.7 Table with built-in back elevator, shown with mattress removed.
1. Back elevator (in raised position)
2. Main control handle (in reversed position)
3. Gear lever
4. Back elevator control
5. Head section quick control
6. Head section fine control

Figure 3.6 continued.
4. Detachable leg section
   (interchangeable with head section)
5. Leg section control
6. Three-position pedal for brake, wheel and castor
7. Height control pedal
8. Main control handle (in retracted position)
9. Gear lever for selecting following positions:
   a. Chair and break
   b. Lateral tilt
   c. Trendelenburg
   d. Extension/flexion
10. Head section quick control
11. Head section fine control

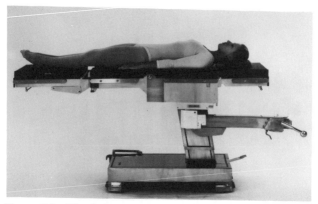

Figure 3.8 The laparotomy or supine position.

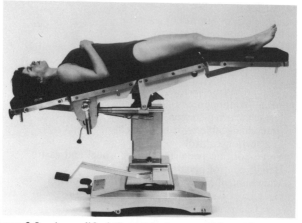

Figure 3.9 A modified Trendelenburg position. The patient's knees are positioned directly over the lower break of the table. The foot of the table can be lowered to flex the knees.

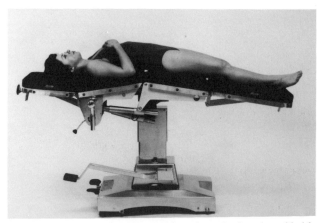

Figure 3.10 These photographs show how the break and bridge in the table may be used for operations on the gallbladder.

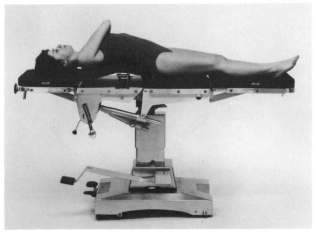

Figure 3.11

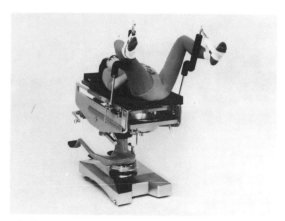

Figure 3.12 The lithotomy position: used for operations on the perineum, anal region and external genital organs. This position can also be modified for use in genito-urinary surgery. Great care should be taken to ensure that both the patient's legs are raised at the same time.

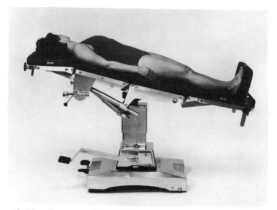

Figure 3.13 Reverse Trendelenburg position, used for operations in the area of the neck.

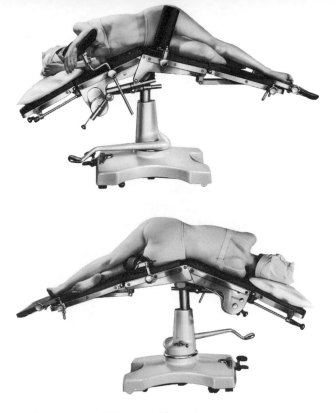

Figure 3.14   The kidney position.

The patient is placed in the lateral position with the affected side upper-most. The underneath leg is fully flexed at the knee, with the foot placed under the uppermost leg. Pads are used to prevent skin friction. The bridge of the table is raised to elevate the loin region between the lower ribs and the iliac crest. The uppermost arm is supported on a padded rest and the underneath arm is pulled a little away from the body and flexed at the elbow with the hand under the patient's face.

This position, but usually without the raised bridge, is used for rib resection, for draining an empyema, and also for thoracoplasty.

The bridge is lowered and the table straightened before muscle sutures are tied.

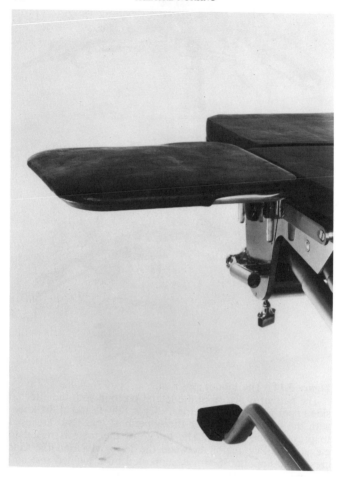

Figure 3.15 This support can be attached to the table for operations on the hand, arm or axilla.

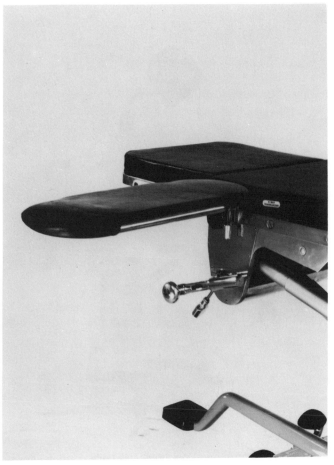

Figure 3.16 This support can be attached to the table to extend the arm for operations on the chest wall.

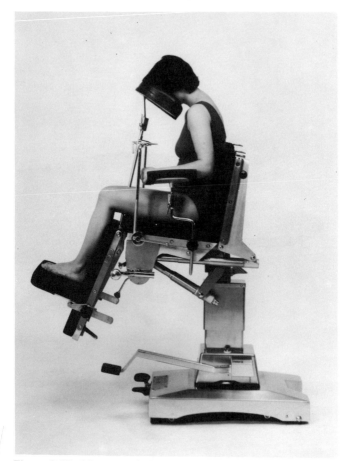

Figure 3.17 Neurosurgical position. This table position allows maximum ease of movement for the surgeon. All the controls are located on the patient's side.

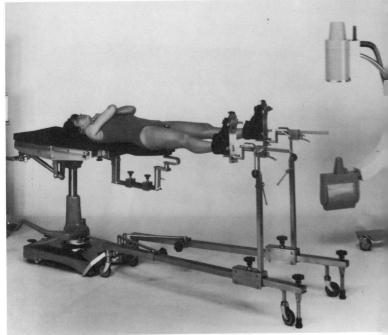

Figure 3.18 Position for orthopaedic procedures of the lower extremities and pelvic girdle. The orthopaedic attachment is designed for use with the image intensifer and with conventional radiography apparatus. The top section of the table is removed before surgery, to allow access for the anaesthetist.

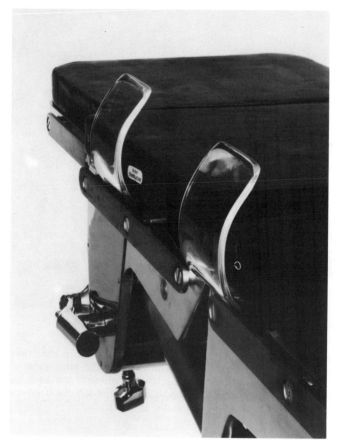

Figure 3.19 Arm supports.

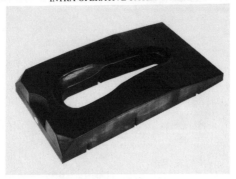

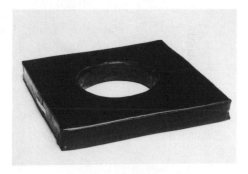

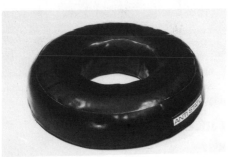

Figure 3.20 A selection of head stabilisers for use in ENT surgery and operations on the head and face.

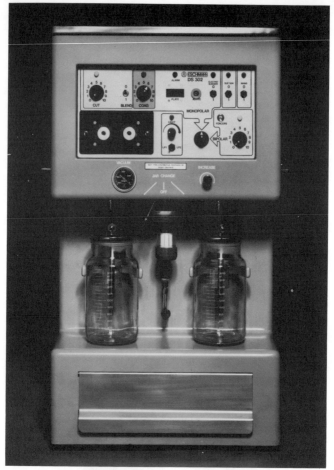

Figure 3.21 Solid-state bipolar and high-power monopolar electro-surgery with suction and fibrelight source.

FURTHER READING

Electrosurgery

Brigden, R.J. (1988) *Operating Theatre Technique*, 5th edn, 'Electricity and electromedical equipment', pp. 67–107, Churchill Livingstone, Edinburgh.

DHSS (1982) 'Evaluation of surgical diathermy units', HEI 99 (April).
DHSS (1982) 'Management of equipment', HEI 98 (Jan.).
DHSS (1982) 'Severe burns caused by chemical action with diathermy plates', *Safety Information Bulletin*, (6) (2 Sept.).
'Evaluation of surgical diathermy units', *Journal Med. Eng. Technol.*, 9(6) (Nov.–Dec. 1985): 281–3.
Health & Safety Executive (1984) Guidance Notes GS27, 'Protection against electric shock'.
Keymed, 'Radio-frequency cutting and coagulation in endoscopic use', Olympus Keymed.
Lieth, I.M. (1980) 'Electrical safety in the hospital', *American Journal of Nursing* (July): 1344–8.
MDU/RCN/NATN (1988) *Theatre Safeguards*.
NATN, (1991) *Principles of Safe Practice in the Operating Department – Resource Book*, NATN, Harrogate, Yorks.
Safety Information Bulletin (1985) 'Loss of diathermy plate monitor function due to defective dry plate electrode holders', 85(3) (Jan.).
Safety Information Bulletin (1987) 'Surgical diathermy avoiding patient burns', 87(66) (Sept.).
Safety Information Bulletin (1988) 'Insulation of bi-polar diathermy dissecting forceps', 88(59) (Sept.).
Wainwright, D. (1988) 'Diathermy: how safe is it?' *British Journal of Theatre Nursing*, 25(1).
Wicker, C.P. (1991) *Working with Electrosurgery*, NATN, Harrogate, Yorks.*

General

Anderton, J.M., Keen, R.I. and Neave, R. (1988) *Positioning the Surgical Patient*, Butterworths, London.*
Brigden, R.J. (1988) *Operating Theatre Techniques (5th Edn)*, Churchill Livingstone, Edinburgh.*
Coombes, B. (1978). 'The importance of being well-dressed in theatre', *Natnews*, 15: 6–8.
Dixon, E. (1985) *The Theatre Nurse and the Law*, Baillière Tindall, London.*
Freidin, J. and Marshall, V. (1984) *Illustrated Guide to Surgical Practice*, Churchill Livingstone, Edinburgh.
Graves, F.T. and Graves, D. (1979) *Seeing Operating Surgery*, Heinemann, London.
MDU, MPS, MDDUS, NATN, RCN (1986) *Theatre Safeguards*.*
NATN, (1991) *Principles of Safe Practice in the Operating Department – a Resource Book*, NATN, Harrogate.*
Nightingale, K. (1987) *Learning to Care in the Theatre*, Hodder & Stoughton, London.*
Warren, M.C. (1983) *Operating Theatre Nursing*, Harper & Row, London.

* Highly recommended

4 Post-operative patient care

INTRODUCTION

From the moment of anaesthetisation until consciousness returns, the patient's safety is the responsibility of health professionals in the operating department.

The recovery room

The term 'recovery room' has many meanings. The functions differ according to particular operating departments and local health policies. In some operating departments a specially designated ward will be available to admit patients to the operating department and to care for them in the immediate post-operative period, whereas in other departments the immediate post-operative care of the patient will take place away from the operating department and back on the surgical ward.

All recovery rooms admit patients immediately after surgery. The length of time the patient remains in the recovery room will be determined by locally agreed protocols for transfer. In some units the stay will be restricted to a few hours, whilst in others it may be two or three days. Recovery rooms tend to be equipped to provide facilities for pre-operative resuscitation, and long-term treatment of artificially ventilated patients. Recovery rooms provide a form of intensive care which is an essential part of peri-operative patient care.

Short-stay post-anaesthetic recovery wards

These have two main advantages for surgical nursing:

1. Such an environment, with appropriately qualified nursing staff, ensures that the post-anaesthetic patient is continuously and adequately cared for in a situation where all the necessary treatment facilities are immediately available.
2. A designated recovery room ensures efficient and effective deployment use of surgical ward staff.

Care of the post-operative patient requires careful observation and planned interventions. The following observations are essential for all patients:

MAINTAINING THE PATIENT'S AIRWAY

Complete respiratory obstruction can lead to death in 3 minutes. It is therefore necessary to check that the patient is breathing by actually feeling air coming out of the patient's mouth or nose. Use the palm of the hand or listen with an ear close to the mouth.

The artificial airway

The most commonly used artificial airway is the Guedel airway, which is made of plastic and is disposable. Occasionally, black rubber Guedel airways are used. These are re-usable.

The Guedel airway facilitates the maintenance of unobstructed breathing, and many patients are transferred to the recovery room with such an airway in place. In a straightforward, uncomplicated recovery from anaesthesia the patient will wake up and remove the airway, either by hand or by spitting it out. Sometimes, a patient will swallow and push the airway slightly forward. It is

important that the nurse leaves the airway in this position
and does not push it back into the patient's throat, as
this will precipitate retching and vomiting.

Very occasionally, it may be necessary to pull away
the airway to a half position if laryngeal spasm occurs,
but generally the airway will remain fully in position until
the patient can respond to a spoken command to open
the mouth.

Causes of an obstructed airway

(a) Tongue falling back
(b) Secretions, i.e. blood, mucus
(c) Vomiting
(d) Foreign body
(e) Compression of artificial airway
(f) Laryngeal spasm
(g) Oedema
(h) Compression of trachea by haematoma.

(a) Tongue falling back

The airway can be obstructed by the tongue falling back
against the wall of the pharynx. If the obstruction is
partial, a snoring noise is produced. If obstruction is
complete, no noise at all is present, but sternal recession
may be visible.

The treatment is to stand behind the patient and pull
the tongue forward by pushing the angles of the jaw
upward and forward. This is usually successful, but the
amount of force required varies considerably. If necessary,
the patient should be positioned laterally. It may be
necessary to use tongue forceps to bring the tongue
forward.

(b) Secretions

The presence of secretions or blood in the airway may be recognised by a 'rattling' sound when the patient breathes. The treatment of this condition is to remove the secretions using suction apparatus, and if necessary, turning the patient on to one side and lowering the head of the trolley or bed.

(c) Vomiting

Vomiting or regurgitation in an unconscious patient requires emergency action for the following reasons. Firstly, the protective laryngeal reflexes are depressed and therefore the patient is at risk of inhaling vomit into the lungs.

Secondly, even though the laryngeal reflexes may not be fully abolished, the associated spasm and breath-holding which occurs can cause severe anoxic strain.

To pre-empt the dangers of vomiting the patient is usually nursed on one side. If signs of vomiting are obvious, then the head of the trolley should be lowered and pharyngeal suction applied to clear the patient's airway. The anaesthetist should also be informed when an anaesthetised patient has vomited.

(d) Foreign body

Occasionally the patient's airway may be obstructed by the presence of a foreign body; e.g. a throat pack which has not been removed or tooth which has been dislodged during intubation. In each case the foreign body must be removed.

(e) Compression of artificial airway

If the Guedel airway is not fully inserted, the patient may bite the curved, soft portion and compress it. To relieve this, apply pressure to the patient's chin in order to open the mouth. Occasionally it may be necessary to use a mouth gag.

(f) Laryngeal spasm

Laryngeal spasm results from direct irritation of the larynx, and in the post-operative period this is usually due to the presence of vomitus, blood or mucus in the patient's airway. Alternatively, particular surgical intervention may predispose towards laryngeal spasm; e.g. following bronchoscopy, or a traumatic endotracheal intubation, especially in children, or patients with chronic bronchitis. The characteristic high-pitched crowing noise heard only on inspiration during laryngeal spasm is referred to as 'stridor'.

If the laryngeal spasm is very severe, it may be necessary for the anaesthetist to administer a muscle relaxant and re-intubate the patient in order to achieve ventilation.

If laryngeal spasm occurs in the post-anaesthetic patient, then the recovery room staff should:

- Obtain medical assistance.
- Turn the patient on to one side and lower the head of the bed or trolley.
- Remove all secretions from the larynx by suction.
- Administer oxygen to ensure optimum air entry via the partly closed glottis.

Very occasionally, laryngeal spasm may be caused by the artificial airway being too long for the patient. If this is suspected, remove the airway about 1/2–1 inch only, administer oxygen and pull the patient's chin forward.

(g) Oedema

After surgery to the mouth, or pharynx or larynx, oedema may develop. This can cause an obstructed airway. If oedema starts to develop, send for medical aid, as a tracheostomy may be necessary.

(h) Compression of trachea by haematoma

This complication may arise after neck surgery; e.g. following thyroidectomy. If the wound edges have been clipped or stapled, these should be removed. Release the haematoma and seek medical assistance urgently.

When caring for any anaesthetised patient, frequently check the patient's airway to ensure adequate oxygenation.

RESPIRATION

Following anaesthesia it is important to observe the rate and depth of respiration. It is vital to watch for signs of respiratory depression; that is, the presence of slow, shallow respirations and possible cyanosis. An important sign of respiratory inadequacy is tracheal tug. This is jerky 'tugging' of the larynx, present with each inspiration. It is often associated with tightening of muscles under the chin and may be due to a partially obstructed airway, a pneumothorax, the persisting effect of muscle relaxant drugs or carbon dioxide retention.

If respiratory inadequacy is present, there is a danger that the patient will retain carbon dioxide. The signs of a raised arterial carbon dioxide level are tachycardia, a rise in blood pressure, sweating and a declining level of consciousness. If these signs are present, then it is essential that the nurse seeks medical assistance and that blood gas analyses are carried out.

For the majority of post-surgical patients oxygen will be administered via a face mask. However, care must be taken in administering oxygen to patients with chronic bronchitis. These patients must be given a low concentration of oxygen via a 'ventimask', as too high a concentration of oxygen may lead to carbon dioxide retention and respiratory failure.

MUSCULAR RIGIDITY

During the immediate post-operative recovery of patients who have received a general anaesthetic, there is a phase when all muscles are contracted. This usually lasts a few minutes only. Sometimes this is accompanied by shivering, which may occasionally become violent. Heat loss during surgery and the use of certain anaesthetic agents predisposes to these phenomena.

When this happens it is important to ensure that the patient's airway does not become obstructed and that the patient does not suffer injury. In all cases of muscle rigidity, with partial airway obstruction, the administration of oxygen hastens the return of muscle relaxation.

As always, attention to the airway is first priority, but if shaking is very violent, it may be necessary to prevent the patient from injury against the sides of the trolley or bed, or, more usually, from disturbing drains and dressings.

RESTLESSNESS

Some transient restlessness is a normal accompaniment to recovery from anaesthesia. Treatment in the first instant is gentle and careful reassurance and orientation of the patient. Restraint should not be used, as this will provoke further struggling by the patient.

This restlessness usually subsides in 10 or 15 minutes, during which time the nurse can assess the cause of the restlessness. In the immediate post-operative situation this may be due to mental confusion, fear or pain. Empathic communication is necessary, and where appropriate an analgesic should be administered.

A more serious cause of restlessness is cerebral hypoxia. This may be associated with partial residual paralysis due to the active presence of muscle-relaxant drugs.

Other causes of restlessness are intra-venous fluid therapy splints which are uncomfortable, wound dressings which are too tight, the pressure of a full bladder or even excessive maintainance of the patient's airway by an inexperienced nurse.

THE CIRCULATION

Many drugs used for premedication and anaesthesia depress, to varying degrees, the compensating vaso-motor reflexes which maintain the normal blood pressure. This means that an anaesthetised patient will tend to have a lower blood pressure than usual, and a less than stable circulation. Sudden and sometimes dangerous falls of blood pressure may result in response to stimuli which at other times would have a negligible effect.

This instability of the circulation is particularly marked in the immediate post-operative period, and the factors most likely to precipitate a circulatory collapse vary considerably. The most obvious are: sudden haemorrhage, hypovolaemia and sudden movement of the patient. In addition, the patient may be at risk following the administration of analgesic drugs, during the syncope of impending vomiting, and anoxia from any cause such as transient holding of the breath and respiratory obstruction.

If it is discovered that the patient has a low blood

pressure (normally defined as a systolic value of 90), then specific actions should be taken. Firstly, the nurse should establish the 'normal' or baseline blood pressure for the patient. Next, the rate of the intravenous infusion should be increased and the foot of the bed or trolley raised and medical assistance sought.

During the recovery period the patient's pulse may change rapidly, both in rate and quality. Any irregularities should, of course, be reported immediately, as should a persistent rise above 110 or fall below 60. A patient with an irregular pulse is usually attached to an electrocardiogram monitor. A not uncommon cause of a very slow pulse is an excessive dose of the drug Prostigmine, which may require the administration of further atropine.

Controlled hypotension

Certain analgesic techniques – e.g. epidural or spinal anaesthetic or the use of ganglion blocking agents, such as Ansolysen (Trimetiphen) – deliberately lower the blood pressure considerably.

Spinal and epidural anaesthesia

When spinal or epidural anaesthetics have been given, the patient's blood pressure will be reduced. Such patients require to be nursed in the supine position, and hypotension may persist after sensation has returned.

SKIN COLOUR

Ideally, the skin of a post-operative patient is 'warm, pink and dry', but there are frequent departures from this state, although most of these changes are transient and short-term.

Recognising cyanosis in the patient who is 'pink' is

relatively easy. Less widely appreciated is the fact that this sign is not obvious in the anaemic patient, and indeed, may never occur if the anaemia is very severe. Conversely, a few plethoric patients are cyanosed even though they are adequately oxygenated. It can also be difficult to detect cyanosis in people with pigmented skin, even by looking at the mucous membranes of the lips, tongue or mouth. In any recovery room it is essential that good lighting is provided to assist with the observation of the patient for cyanosis.

For all these reasons, emphasis must be laid on the care of the airway and the prevention of anoxia, rather than on detecting cyanosis alone.

In fit patients cyanosis is not usually noticeable until after the airway has been obstructed for some time. In all ill patients, however, this interval is very much shorter or may not exist at all. Confusion occasionally arises when a patient who appears otherwise well, with full, unobstructed respiration and normal pulse and blood pressure, is yet a little blue around the lips and cheeks. The situation may be clarified if these areas are gently rubbed. If they turn pink there is no cause for alarm, but if not, oxygen must be given.

PALLOR

While extreme pallor indicates exsanguination, anaemia or 'shock', it is not uncommon for patients to become pale during recovery from anaesthesia. If the pulse and blood pressure – and of course, the respiration – are within normal limits, there is no cause for alarm, but if the blood pressure is low, then nursing interventions should be instigated.

EYES

Care of the eyes is of importance in patients recovering from anaesthesia, as in all unconscious patients. It is all too easy to push an eye open when turning a patient onto his side or the semi-prone position, or when the lower eye is buried in the pillow. It is even easier inadvertently to open and damage an eye with a face mask, as when giving artificial respiration with the ambu-bag. The treatment is simple; close the eye if there is a possibility of this mishap. Very occasionally it will be necessary to strap the eyes shut.

The clinical signs shown by the eyes in patients recovering from anaesthesia are complex, and only widely dilated pupils which do not react to light need cause concern. Such dilated pupils are observed in cases of cardiac arrest, head injury and some neurosurgical interventions or X-ray procedures. If the pupils are dilated, then it is important that the pupil reactions and sizes are recorded and documented at regular intervals.

Widely dilated pupils, however, may also be seen after ganglion blocking drugs have been given to lower blood pressure, or when the premedication consisted of atropine alone. These are normal responses, but the former cause is a reminder that the circulation is still likely to be sensitive to movement and postural changes.

PRESSURE AREAS

The care of pressure areas is, of course, one of the fundamentals of nursing care. It is, however, worth remembering that these areas are particularly at risk in the recovery ward for three reasons:

- Many patients will be hypotensive, hence reducing the blood supply to those parts.

- During the period of restlessness, patients can easily come to be in an unsatisfactory position, on a 'rucked' canvas.
- The pressure points have already been subjected to unnatural prolonged pressure whilst the patient was lying on the operating table.

Pressure areas should be checked regularly and preventative aids used as appropriate, e.g. sheepskin heel muffs, special mattresses.

TEMPERATURE CONTROL

It will be necessary to record a patient's temperature in the recovery ward, especially for those individuals who have undergone operations under hypothermia, or patients who have had or are having a blood transfusion, or if the patient is to remain in the recovery ward for a long period of time. If after long, major operations, recovery is prolonged, a sub-normal temperature may occur. Elderly patients and children are susceptible to high degrees of heat loss. No treatment is usually indicated beyond preventing further heat loss with the use of special heat-retaining blankets. On the other hand, hyperpyrexia is abnormal, and the patient should be cooled immediately by exposure and the use of air circulating fans.

Sweating

This may be due to high temperature, but may also be the result of inadequate ventilation, retention of carbon dioxide and post-operative analgesic drugs.

HEARING

Just as a sense of hearing is the last sensation to be
abolished during the induction of anaesthesia, so it is the
first to return during recovery. This means that many
apparently unconscious patients, including some with
artificial airways in their mouths, can hear and remember
words spoken around them, even though they may be
confused about the time and place. The importance of
careful expression and comment under these circumstances is well known – but particular care should be
taken in the recovery room.

IDENTIFICATION

Particular care is required by the nurse to identify the
patient. Frequently, in large operating departments more
than one patient will arrive in the recovery room at the
same time. The name of the patient, the operation
performed, the theatre and the ward the patient has come
from, any special instructions regarding care and the
names of surgeons and anaesthetists concerned must
always be ascertained immediately on admission to the
recovery ward.

PAIN CONTROL

In the recovery room the control of the pain experiences
of the patient is of importance. There are many methods
of pain control deployed nowadays. The most common
is still the intra-muscular injection of an opiate alkaloid.
Drugs such as Morphine sulphate, Papaveretum and
Pethidine are widely used.

The use of local anaesthetics into the operating
site during surgery also has an analgesic effect post-

operatively, as does the use of epidural or spinal anaesthetics.

The use of cryo-surgical techniques for post-operative pain relief following thoracotomy has been popular in recent years. More recently, infusions of analgesics controlled by patients has become a recognised method of pain control. TENS electrodes placed along wound edges have also been effective in reducing pain experiences.

Although pain experiences have a physiological and biochemical base, the amount of discomfort felt by an individual is subjective, and the nurse should always respond to a patient's request for pain relief.

CARDIO-PULMONARY RESUSCITATION

In each recovery room there will be resuscitation equipment. This is usually a self-contained mobile trolley with an integral stand for supporting intravenous infusions, equipment drawers, a cardiac board and working surface. All resuscitation trolleys have electrical sockets and are generally connected to the mains supply to ensure that the defibrillator remains charged.

The following range of equipment may be housed on an adult resuscitation trolley.

On the working surface

Defibrillator with long-life electrodes and adult paddles attached electrolyte gel, tissues and spare ECG electrodes.

Most modern defibrillators have built in ECG monitors and display units. However, if these are not integral to the defibrillator, an ECG monitor should also be available.

First drawer – endotracheal equipment

1. Macintosh laryngoscope with interchangeable adult blades.
2. Spare bulb and long-life batteries for laryngoscope.
3. Magill forceps (adult size).
4. Mouthgag with Acklands Jaws.
5. Spencer Wells forceps 12.7 cm (5″).
6. Scissors (blunt ends).
7. Neoplex or gum elastic bougie 9 and 14 FG.
8. Syringe for inflating ET tube.
9. Endotracheal tubes, sizes 7.0, 8.0 and 9.00 m (sterile, disposable, oral cuffed with 15 m adaptor).
10. Endotracheal tube catheter mounts (one disposable and one with suction port).
11. 'Satin slip' stylet for endotracheal tubes.
12. Disposable scalpel handle with size 10 blade.
13. Adhesive tape 2.5 cm (1″).
14. Gauze swabs 7.5 cm (3″).
15. KY jelly.
16. Assorted intra-cardiac needles.

Second drawer – intravenous equipment

1. 'Venflon' IV cannulae – 2 each of 14, 16, 17 and 20 gauge.
2. Assorted Quickcaths.
3. Filling cannulae × 3.
4. Syringes – 2 ml, 5 ml, 10 ml and 20 ml.
5. Hypodermic needles, 21, 23 and 25 gauge.
6. Medicated swabs.
7. Sterile, disposable 3-way luer locking taps × 2.
8. Adhesive tape 2.5 cm (1″).
9. Gauze swabs 7.5 cm (3″).
10. Assorted Butterfly cannulae.

Third drawer – intravenous fluids and intra-cardiac equipment

1. Recipient sets for blood transfusion × 2 plus Air-inlets.
2. Vygon Leader Catheter, size 14 FG.
3. Sterile, disposable thoracic trocar and cannulae, sizes 24 and 36 FG.
4. Sodium bicarbonate 4.2% w/v 500 ml × 3.
5. Dextrose 5% w/v 500 ml × 1.
6. Dextran 6% w/v 70 injection BP in normal saline 500 ml × 1.
7. Sodium chloride injection 0.9% w/v 500 ml × 1.
8. Mannitol 20% w/v × 1 500 ml × 1.
9. Compound Sodium lactate injection VP 500 ml × 1.
10. Drug box containing range of '3rd Line' intravenous and intracardiac drugs.
11. Sterile chest intubation and thoracotomy pack.
12. Sterile internal defibrillation paddles and cable.
13. Mini tracheostomy kit.

CARDIAC DEFIBRILLATION

When working in the recovery room it is important that the nurse becomes familiar with and competent in the use of resuscitation equipment.

If the resuscitation trolley is required, unplug the trolley from the mains socket and walk briskly with the trolley to the place of cardiac arrest. Where possible, reconnect the trolley to the electrical mains. Raise the intravenous fluid support, and use either for fluids or emergency drugs. If intubation equipment is needed, locate the appropriate laryngoscope and endotracheal tube.

Switch on the defibrillator and prepare the paddles with electrolyte gel. Place the prepared paddles on the

Table 4.1   Drugs for cardiac arrest

Drug	Effect and Dosage
Adrenaline	Causes peripheral vasoconstriction. 1 ml 1:10 000. An increase in pulse rate and myocardial contractility.
Calcium gluconate	Used to increase the strength of cardiac muscle contraction. 10 ml/10%.
Atropine sulphate	Increase heart rate by blocking vagal stimulation. 0.6 mg.
Aminophylline	Is a bronchodilator and also increases myocardial contractility. 250 mg/10 ml.
Lignocaine	Used after treatment of ventricular fibrillation if the rhythm which returns is either ventricular tachycardia or runs of ventricular ectopics as it depresses myocardial excitability. 50–100 mg.
Hydrocortisone	Helps maintain blood pressure after allergic reaction.
Sodium bicarbonate	Used to correct metabolic acidosis. 8.4%. 4.2%.
Frusemide	Diuretic, helps keep kidneys flushed, and if patient has previous severe cardiac failure. 50 mg/5 ml.

patient. One paddle is placed to the right of the sternum, the other paddle goes under the left nipple. In many modern defibrillators this action will provide an ECG tracing of the patient's heart rhythm on the defibrillator monitor. Otherwise, apply ECG electrodes and attach to a separate monitor.

Ask medical staff for the charge setting. For the average adult this tends to be 200–300 joules for external defibrillation. Charge the paddles, using either the charge button on the Apical paddle or the charge button on the front of the defibrillating machine.

The discharge buttons are located on the top of the paddles. A member of the medical staff discharges the paddles by pressing discharge buttons simultaneously. ENSURE THAT NO MEMBER OF STAFF IS IN CONTACT WITH THE PATIENT OR THE OPERATING TABLE/TROLLEY/BED when the DISCHARGE buttons are pressed. A verbal warning to STAND CLEAR should be given prior to DISCHARGING THE DEFIBRILLATOR.

If further external defibrillations are required, clean the patient's chest and the paddles of electrolyte gel, re-apply fresh gel to the paddles and proceed as above.

INTERNAL DEFIBRILLATION

If it is necessary to open the patient's chest, an emergency thoracotomy pack should be located on the trolley along with specially designed internal paddles and connecting cable. Disconnect the external paddle cable and connect the internal paddle cable. Place the paddles around the patient's heart, charge the paddles (5–60 joules for an adult) and discharge the paddles using the thumb switch on one of the paddle handles.

FURTHER READING

Ayers, C. and Walton, L. (1974) 'A guide for the pre-operative visit', *Journal of American Operating Room Nurses*, 19: 413–18.

Boore, J.R.P. (1978) *Prescription for Recovery*, RCN, London.*

Burnett, J. (1988) Unpublished teaching handouts, G1–8 Theatres, Aberdeen Royal Infirmary.

Dinniaio, M.J. and Ingoldsbry, B. (1983) 'Parental presence in the recovery room', *Journal of American Operating Room Nurses*, 38: 685.*

Faulkner, A. (ed.) (1984) *Recent Advances in Nursing Communication*, Churchill Livingstone, Edinburgh.

Frost, A.M. (1985) *Recovery Room Practice*, Blackwell Scientific Publications, Oxford.*

Gruendeman, B.J., Casterton, S., Hesterley, S., Munckley, B.B. and Shetler, M.G. (1973) *The Surgical Patient: Behavioural Concepts for the Operating Room Nurse*, C.V. Mosby, St Louis, MO.

Hunt, J. and Marks Maran, D. (1980) *Nursing Care Plans*, H.M. & M. Publishers, Aylesbury, Bucks.

Johnston, I.D.A. and Hunter, A.R. (eds) (1985) *The Design and Utilisation of Operating Theatres*, Arnold, London.

Kanda, N.L. (1977) 'Staff Development for R.R. Nurses', *Journal of American Operating Room Nurses* 26: 664–7.

Lang, R. (1981) *Systematic Nursing Care*, Faber & Faber, London.

MDU, MPS, MDDUS, NATN, RCN (1986) *Theatre Safeguards*.

NATN (1991) *Principles of Safe Practice in the Operating Department – a Resource Book*, NATN, Harrogate.

Nightingale, K. (1987) *Learning to Care in the Theatre*, Hodder & Stoughton, London.*

Ostler, G. and Bryce-Smith, R. (1982) *Anaesthetics for Medical Students*, Churchill Livingstone, Edinburgh.

Ridgway, M. (1976) 'Preop interviews assure quality care', *Journal of American Operating Room Nurses*, 2: 1083.

Schmidt, F.E. and Woolridge, P.J. (1973) 'Psychological preparation of surgical patients', *NURS Res.* (March/April): 108–15.

Smith, C.E. (1978) 'Planning, implementing and evaluating learning experiences for adults', *Nurse Educator* (Nov.–Dec.).

The Misuse of Drugs (Safe Custody Regulations (1973)).The Health and Safety at Work Act (1974) Part I, Section I, HMSO, London.

Utting, J.E. (1985) 'Anaesthetic aspects: the anaesthetic and recovery rooms', in I.D.A. Johnston and A.R. Hunter (eds) *The Design and Utilisation of Operating Theatres*, Arnold, London.

Vance, J.P. and Corrigan, A. (1983) *Post-operative Care*, Heinemann, London.

Wachstein, J. and Smith, J.A.H. (1981) *Anaesthesia and Recovery Room Techniques*, Baillière Tindall, London.

* Highly recommended

5 Models of nursing and care planning

A nursing model can be defined as a collection of ideas and concepts which describes in theoretical terms the elements of nursing care. Models provide a framework around which nurses can plan patient care. There are many models of nursing. In any practice setting it is essential that the nurse selects an appropriate model to suit the clinical environment.

THE SELF-CARE MODEL

This model was developed by Dorothea Orem, and is based on two types of self-care and how nurses can assess any self-care deficits in patients and plan nursing interventions accordingly. This model is particularly useful for theatre nurses involved in day surgery, where discharge planning and the emphasis on self-care is very important.

The first type of self-care is called *'universal self-care'*. This consists of the actions that all human beings carry out, and these are categorised as follows:

1. Maintenance of air, food and water. Each of these is essential to life, growth, development and the repair of body tissue.
2. The process of excretion. As life continues, the human body processes food and oxygen and produces waste materials which need to be excreted.

3. Maintenance of a balance between activity and rest. For the human body to function well, certain levels of activity and rest are required.
4. Maintenance of a balance between solitude and social interaction. Normal human development requires periods of being alone and also periods of interaction with others.
5. Prevention of hazards to human life and well-being. This involves the avoidance of conditions or situations which threaten or endanger the life of the individual.
6. The maintenance of behaviour, health, well-being and lifestyle that are perceived to be within normal limits. Most individuals conform to what is considered to be socially and culturally acceptable.

The second type of self-care is what Orem terms *'health deviation self-care'*. When any person undergoes changes in physical functioning or behaviour, or ability to carry out activities of living, extra demands are made by that person. What causes these changes may be attributed to disease or injury, or alternatively from medical intervention such as surgery.

Therefore, when this deviation in normal self-care abilities takes place, the person can either make up the amount of self-care needed personally, or else seek some kind of intervention. In the case of surgical patients, this intervention is usually nursing care.

The nurse may compensate wholly or partly for the self-care of the patient, or educate and develop the patient in order to assist the patient to achieve full self-care.

THE ACTIVITIES OF LIVING MODEL

This model was developed in the United Kingdom by Nancy Roper, Winifred Logan and Alison Tierney in

1980. They identified activities of living common to all people. These are as follows:

1. Maintaining a safe environment.
2. Communicating.
3. Breathing.
4. Eating and drinking.
5. Eliminating.
6. Personal cleansing and dressing.
7. Controlling body temperature.
8. Mobilising.
9. Working and playing.
10. Expressing sexuality.
11. Sleeping.
12. Dying.

These activities of living are complex and interrelated. During some periods of the hospitalisation of the surgical patient some of these activities cannot be performed. The nurse must adequately assess and prioritise nursing interventions so as to assist the patient with particular activities of living.

This model is useful for planning care for the majority of adult surgical patients, as it enables care to be planned along a continuum of independence. The ward based care plan can therefore be continued in detail in the operating department.

PRIMARY NURSING

Primary nursing is designed to assist with individualised patient care. It is both a philosophy of care and a method of work organisation. The use of a primary nursing approach to care enables the nurse to use whichever model of care best suits the patient and the environment. Primary nursing provides the ideal vehicle for the nursing process, as it allows an individual nurse to assess, plan, implement and evaluate the care of a specific case-load of patients. Primary nursing allows all primary nurses to be responsible and accountable for their own actions.

In addition to managing their own work, primary nurses also manage that of their associate nurses. Ideally, the primary nurse will work exclusively with a personal case-load of patients and has 24-hour responsibility for care. In consultation with the patient the primary nurse plans and evaluates the care, and whilst on duty delivers the planned care; when off duty this planned care is delivered by the associate nurse. The associate nurse may add to the care plan and should discuss changes with the primary nurse at the earliest opportunity.

This method of nursing is particularly useful where the primary nurse from the surgical ward accompanies the patient to the operating department and cares for him or her in the recovery room. It is also useful in situations where the theatre primary nurse carries out pre-operative visiting of the patient, cares for the patient in the anaesthetic room and recovers the patient post-operatively. Primary nursing in the operating department enables the nurse to become involved in holistic patient care.

CARE PLANNING: PATIENT PROBLEMS FREQUENTLY ENCOUNTERED IN THE OPERATING DEPARTMENT

Using the model of Activities of Living (AL), for the majority of adult surgical patients, it is possible to identify the following problems.

Table 5.1

Activity of Living	Patient Problem
Communication	*Fear* related to potential outcome of surgery. For most patients an operation is a daunting event, full of fears about the outcome and success of the operation. The role of the nurse in giving information and reassurance is essential to the patient's psychological well-being.
Dying	*Anticipatory grieving* due to loss of part of the body. Regardless of which part of the body is to be lost, an individual will experience some form of grieving. This grieving process is most pronounced in surgical patients about to undergo mutilating surgery, e.g. mastectomy, amputation of a limb, extensive bowel surgery. Recognition of this process of grieving and the giving of advice to patients and their families about the normal course of events is an important part of nursing care.
Eating and drinking	*Alteration in nutrition.* The process of fasting for surgery will necessarily alter the patient's nutritional status. Because in some cases this may exacerbate a previous chronic condition of malnourishment, it is essential that this is assessed and major deficits or imbalances addressed.
Maintaining a safe environment	*Potential fluid volume deficit.* The process of fasting for surgery will have altered the patient's electrolyte and fluid balance. Furthermore, because the nature of the proposed surgery may result in extensive fluid loss, preventive measures such as pre-operative intravenous infusions may be instigated.

Table 5.1 Continued

Activity of Living	Patient Problem
Sleeping	*Sleep pattern disturbance.* Research studies have shown that the majority of patients in hospital do not sleep well due to unfamiliar surroundings, anxiety about personal health and noise. For the surgical patient the night before an operation may be fraught. It is therefore necessary to support and inform the patient and where necessary administer a previously prescribed sedative or hypnotic.
Maintaining a safe environment	*Anticipatory anxiety* due to unfamiliar environment and impending surgery. This is most marked in the reception area of the operating department or the anaesthetic room. If the nurse can inform the patient in advance of what to expect, and if the physical environment is made comfortable, then the patient's feelings of stress will be minimised.

The pre-operative phase

Patient problems which are common to many adult surgical patients during the pre-operative phase are shown in Table 5.1.

The intra-operative phase

Problems which are common to many adult surgical patients during the intra-operative phase are shown in Table 5.2.

Table 5.2

Activity of living	*Patient problem*
Breathing	*Potential alterations in respiratory function*, due to anaesthesia. This requires the nurse to be aware of normal limits and to monitor the patient's respirations appropriately.
Maintaining a safe environment	*Potential fluid volume deficit*, due to blood loss during surgery. This requires that an accurate record of blood loss during surgery be maintained and recorded. A protocol for maximum levels of blood is useful and a recognised regimen for replacement fluids is available.
Maintaining a safe environment	*Potential for injury*, due to decreased level of consciousness. This requires the nurse to assess, plan and record the positioning of the patient, the movement of an unconscious patient, and the safety precautions to be used with specific equipment, e.g. electrosurgery.
Mobilising	*Potential decrease in cardiac output*, due to anaesthesia, decreased mobility and venous pooling. This requires the nurse to assess the patient for positioning and the most appropriate type of venous stimulation during surgery, and to apply venous stimulation without causing damage to tissue.
Maintaining a safe environment	*Potential for infection*. This requires the nurse to assess, plan, implement and evaluate the aseptic techniques used with each patient, and to ensure a clean, safe environment.

Table 5.3

Activity of living	Patient problem
Mobilising	*Pain* related to surgical incision. This requires the nurse to assess pain experiences objectively through monitoring, and subjectively from patient's accounts, and to act in accordance with medical prescriptions or nursing orders in alleviating pain and reducing restlessness.
Maintaining a safe environment	*Potential injury*, due to returning level of consciousness. This requires the nurse to assess the patient's consciousness level, and to ensure that the immediate environment is safe and remains so.
Breathing	*Ineffective airway clearance*, due to retained secretions. This requires the nurse to assess the respiratory function of the patient, to take preventive actions as appropriate, and to elicit medical assistance if necessary.
Maintaining a safe environment	*Sensory-perceptual alterations*, due to returning level of consciousness. These require that the nurse orientate the patient to time, place and event. Prior warning of the potential for post-operative confusion helps alleviate these problems.

The post-operative phase

Patient problems which are common to the immediate post-operative phase are shown in Table 5.3.

Topic for discussion

Consider the following case history and outline the peri-operative nursing care required using the Roper Logan and Tierney (1980) model of nursing.

A young woman, 24 years old, is admitted to the operating department for surgery. She has acute abdominal pain and is to undergo an emergency laparoscopy and further surgery as required. Her vital signs on admission are:

Temperature	37.6°
Pulse	106
Blood Pressure	140/90
Respirations	20

FURTHER READING

Ayers, C. and Walton, L. (1974) 'A guide for the pre-operative visit', *AORN*, f. 19: 413–18.

Boore, J.R.P. (1978) *Prescription for Recovery*, RCN, London.*

Dinniaio, M.J. and Ingoldsbry, B. (1983) 'Parental presence in the recovery room', *AORN J.*, 38: 685.

Faulkner, A. (ed.) (1984) *Recent Advances in Nursing Communication*, Churchill Livingstone, Edinburgh.

Frost, A.M. (1985) *Recovery Room Practice*, Blackwell Scientific Publications, Oxford.

Greundeman, B.J. et al. (1973) *The Surgical Patient: Behavioural Concepts for the Operating Room Nurse*, C.V. Mosby, St Louis, MO.

Hunt, J. and Marks Maran, D. (1980) *Nursing Care Plans*, H.M. & M. Publishers, Aylesbury, Bucks.

Lang, R. (1981) *Systematic Nursing Care*, Faber & Faber, London.

Nightingale, K. (1987) *Learning to Care in the Theatre*, Hodder & Stoughton, London.

Orem, D.E. (1980) *Nursing: Concepts of Practice*, McGraw-Hill Co., New York (2nd edn).

Ridgway, M. (1976) 'Preop interviews assure quality care', *AORN J.* 2: 1083.

---

*Highly recommended

112 THEATRE NURSING

Roper, W., Logan, W.W. and Tierney, A.J. (1980) *The Elements of Nursing*, Churchill Livingstone, Edinburgh.

Roy, C. (1976) *Introduction to Nursing: an Adaptation Model*, Prentice-Hall, Englewood Cliffs, NJ.

Schmidt, F.E. and Woolridge, P.J. (1973) 'Psychological preparation of surgical patients', *NURS Res*. (March/April): 108–15.

Vance, J.P. and Corrigan, A. (1983) *Post-operative Care*, Heinemann, London.

Wachstein, J. and Smith, J.A.H. (1981) *Anaesthesia and Recovery Room Techniques*, Baillière Tindall, London.

6 Legal and ethical aspects of nursing care in the operating department

This chapter is designed to introduce the student to various legal and ethical aspects of surgical nursing. At the end of the chapter, a case study is presented for self-reflection and/or discussion.

The changing environment, technological advances and developments within nursing generally have resulted in the extension of the role of the theatre nurse. Consequently, all theatre nurses require to be aware of individual responsibility and accountability to the patient. The United Kingdom Central Council Code of Professional Conduct specifies the principles of responsibility and accountability for all qualified nurses, and should be upheld in all aspects of practice.

ACCOUNTABILITY

According to the Code of Professional Conduct, all nurses are accountable for their own practice, and in exercising professional accountability should act in a responsible way towards patients, peers, the profession, other health professionals and society as a whole.

PATERNALISM

Individuals with a strong religious or ideological conviction
may feel that they know what is best for another person.
However, by deciding for that person what is best they
are in principle denying that person's individuality.
This paternalistic approach has been prevalent and has
characterised nurse–patient relationships in the past.

THE NURSING PROCESS

Over the last decade the trend in surgical nursing has
been towards involving the patient in care and decision
making. The nursing process enables the family and the
patient to be involved and to exercise their rights. Within
the nursing process the nurse is encouraged to perceive
and relate to patients as individuals with basic human
needs and particular personal needs. Furthermore, the
patient has rights to contribute to the decision-making
process.

From the patient's perspective this is a good thing, and
in recent years patients' rights movements and the
development of patients' charters have been focal. Once
patients in hospital are treated as individuals, they expect
to have the same rights as any individual and perhaps
some more because they are patients.

From the nurses' perspective this means that the patient
has a right to challenge decisions and treatment. This in
turn may lead to nurses' examining standards of care or
acting as an advocate for the patient.

DUTY

The duty of a qualified nurse is to use knowledge and
skills to maintain expected and reasonable standards of

care. In this connection the nurse has a sense of duty towards self, the patient, professional colleagues and the employer.

Duty to self

The nurse's duty to self involves self-preservation and professional competence. This means that the nurse must not take foolish or rash risks and must be observant, reliable, honest, accurate and gentle. Furthermore, there is an onus of personal and professional responsibility on each nurse to develop positively the skills of caring, teaching and management necessary for relating to professional colleagues and caring for patients within the operating department.

Duty to patients

Whilst in the operating department the patient, who is vulnerable and socially isolated in this strange environment, requires particular compassion and thought. Although most nurses recognise the major ethical or legal concerns regarding the rights and wrongs of administering certain drugs or in carrying out certain procedures, it is also imperative that they consider the ethics of everyday nurse–patient interactions, such as maintaining the patient's dignity during induction of anaesthesia, expressing courtesy when visiting patients pre-operatively, or in supporting conscious patients during surgical procedures, and in informing patients accurately about procedures carried out whilst they are in the operating department.

CULTURAL FACTORS

In a multi-cultural class society certain cultural, religious, social and economic differences can complicate health care. The nurse will have values and norms which are personal and may conflict with professional values. Similarly, the patient may have personal values that are in conflict with nursing or medical values. It is essential therefore that information is available in the operating department on such issues in order that the individual patient care provided does not contradict particular beliefs – e.g. Hindu, Islamic and Jewish beliefs and those of some Christian sects (such as Jehovah's Witnesses or Christian Scientists).

STIGMA

Professional attitudes towards health care and specific illnesses may directly affect patients. Nursing care in the operating department requires expert knowledge which encompasses both technical and psychological aspects of care. In order to address problems of nurses' attitudes and beliefs about specific illnesses it is necessary that open discussions take place and education is available to inform nurses about particular patient groups who have been stigmatised by society generally. For example, hepatitis B patients, HIV patients, patients with self-inflicted injuries and certain ethnic groups have all been subject to stereotyping and stigma.

QUALITY AND SANCTITY OF LIFE

Views on the quality and sanctity of life are usually discussed with regard to major decisions about life and death such as 'Do not resuscitate' orders or abortion. However, there are many issues that may arise in the operating department which affect the quality or sanctity of the patient's life. Just as nurses have professional and ethical codes of conduct, so do other health professionals.

The dilemmas faced by doctors and nurses when faced with the decision to prolong life need careful consideration. Formerly, those arguing for quantity of life believed that *all* life was of equal value. Proponents of quality of life believe that *no* life at all is better than a life with significant deficiencies. Making decisions based on quality of life is difficult because of the absence of criteria for determining quality and the subjective judgements involved. Professional codes of conduct and legislation are essential and are the guiding rules for decision making.

In nursing, value judgements are often made. In the operating theatre many nurses are faced with dilemmas because personal and professional values conflict. In order to enhance the worth of both personal and professional judgements the nurse must aim for excellence in performance, honesty, integrity and an objective consideration of other people's perspectives.

CONSENT

The need for *informed consent* applies to participation in research and participation in *all* nursing or medical procedures carried out on a patient.

Patients have the right to withhold or give consent to treatment. Once embarked upon a course of treatment or involvement in research, the patient also has the right to withdraw. In order, however, for patients to make such judgements it is necessary to provide sufficient information. It is important that the patient receives such information in an easily understood language and in sufficient detail so as to be able to make an educated and informed decision.

Where a surgical patient is unable to provide consent – such as in the situation of an unconscious patient requiring life-saving surgery – then someone else has to make that decision. This may be a relative or, if the situation warrants, then the surgeon is justified in making the decision in the best interests of the patient.

Where a minor is involved in surgery, the consent of the parent or guardian is sought. The same rights of informed and educated consent prevail, and the nurse will wish to assist the parents in informing the child of the surgery in such a way as to alleviate anxiety and fear.

CONFIDENTIALITY

Within the operating department the patient has a right to confidentiality and the nurse has a duty to uphold that right. In the operating theatre nurses are often in possession of information which may cause distress if divulged to others. Information revealed at the time of operation is strictly confidential and should not be discussed with others.

The patient's medical and nursing notes are confidential and therefore accessible to scrutiny by authorised personnel only, and must always remain with the patient. Where patient records are computerised and displayed on a Visual Display Unit within the operating department, it is necessary that precautions are taken to prevent perusal of this information by unauthorised individuals.

WRITTEN RECORDS

The patient's right to see medical and nursing records is now upheld by law. The theatre nurse is responsible for keeping accurate and legible records which are reliable and accessible. All operating departments will have an Operating Theatre Register which is used to record details of all patients receiving surgery, the nature of the surgery and the names of the operating team involved.

With the Consumer Protection Act certain information pertaining to products used during surgery will also be recorded.

NURSING CARE PLANS

The nurse has a responsibility to record the peri-operative care of the patient. This should be accurate and comprehensive, and should cover the pre-, intra- and post-operative phases of care. The information recorded is confidential and pertinent to the care of the patient whilst in the operating department.

NEGLIGENCE

Negligence can be defined as the failure to exercise the care which can be reasonably expected of a nurse in certain circumstances. In order to prove negligence in law it is essential to establish the following:

- That duty of care was owed by the nurse to the patient.
- That the nurse did not carry out that duty.
- That as a result, damage was caused or the patient was harmed.

In addition, negligence can be defined as 'culpable negligence', where a responsible person delegates to another tasks or aspects of care that the delegated person is not capable of carrying out or qualified to perform.

Finally, failure to report an incident can also be considered as negligence if suffering or harm is caused. Each of these definitions of negligence places an onus of responsibility on the nurse, who is responsible legally and ethically for his or her own conduct, in carrying out instructions or querying them if they are considered neither reasonable nor safe.

Safeguards

Safeguards against wrong operations being performed or foreign bodies being left inside patients at the time of surgery have been considered by the professional bodies representing doctors and nurses. Joint recommendations for procedures to prevent wrong operations and failure to remove foreign bodies have been developed by the National Association of Theatre Nurses, the Royal College of Nursing and the Medical Defence Union.

RESEARCH

There are guidelines on the ethics of research set out by the Royal College of Nursing. Within these guidelines there are clear recommendations concerning consent, the value of the research, the risk–benefit ratio, the mutual obligations of the researcher and the sponsor of the research, and the role of the researcher in the workplace.

Any research carried out in the operating department must be necessary and contribute to further knowledge. Prior to commencing research, it is essential that all research proposals are vetted and approved by a local Ethical Committee. Most Health Authorities, Health Boards and Hospital Trusts have Ethical Committees which are convened regularly throughout the year. These committees are composed of experts and lay members. Generally, the nursing profession, the major branches of medicine, the legal profession and the clergy are represented on such committees.

TOPIC FOR DISCUSSION

Consider the following case study and discuss the ethical and legal implications of the actions involved.

Background and complaint

The patient was admitted to hospital on 29 August 1979 for the birth of her child. On the following day it was decided to perform a Caesarean section, and serious problems were encountered during intubation. After the operation the patient was transferred to the high dependency unit whilst her baby daughter spent some time in the special care baby unit.

When the patient was told that she required a Caesarean section she informed the surgeon, midwife and theatre nurse that she couldn't be intubated. She recalled that the surgeon made no response to this but busied himself apparently either reading or making notes. When she arrived in theatre the anaesthetic registrar spoke to her while she was on the trolley and said he understood that there had been some difficulty previously. The patient replied that this was so and that the information was all in the notes from 1973. The anaesthetic registrar reassured her and promised to take great care.

The anaesthetic registrar said that it was not unusual in the event of an emergency Caesarean section for the anaesthetist not to see the patient before her arrival in theatre. In attempting to intubate her he grazed the back of her throat and decided that he would have to waken her. He did so and she started to breathe spontaneously, but at this stage she suffered laryngo-spasm and he was unable to ventilate her.

At the same time the nurse could not feel her pulse at the wrist and the registrar could not feel a carotid pulse. He called for the resuscitation trolley and during this time the complainant became blue. The cardiac arrest routine was implemented and, although the anaesthetist did not ask for it, the nurse started to give external cardiac massage on his own initiative. After 30 seconds the anaesthetic registrar was able to ventilate the patient. On examining the clinical and nursing notes relating to this period in the anaesthetic room it was seen that the surgeon, the midwife and the anaesthetic nurse had recorded that the patient had suffered a cardiac arrest before intubation in their respective notes.

Immediately following the section the baby made some efforts to breathe, but these were inadequate and her heart rate was failing. Because of that the baby was intubated and ventilated until 7 minutes after birth. She was cold and remained pale and was transferred to the special care baby unit where a blood gas test showed some degree of acidosis.

Consequently the patient lodged the following complaints:

(a) The patient contended that her life and that of her baby were put at unnecessary risk because conclusions which had been reached in 1973 about intubating her were not included in her medical history in her obstetric notes.

(b) She said that the 1973 medical notes were not called for at any time and complained that even though she gave information about the findings to two doctors, a midwife and a nurse before the operation, it was ignored.

(c) The complainant also said that in subsequent correspondence the assistant general administrator of the hospital unreasonably minimised the risk to her and her daughter.

Adapted and modified from *Report of the Health Service*

Commissioner: Selected Investigations Completed April 1983–September 1983 and April 1982–September 1982, HMSO, London. Case No. 2 No. W.241/ 79–80– Availability of Mother's Previous Medical History to an Anaesthetist prior to Delivery of a Baby by Caesarean Section.

FURTHER READING

Benjamin, M. (1986) *Ethics in Nursing*, Oxford University Press, Oxford.

Dixon, E. (1984) *The Theatre Nurse and the Law*, Croom Helm, London.

Burnard, P. and Chapman, M.M. (1988) *Professional and Ethical Issues in Nursing*, Wiley and Sons, Chichester.

Fitzpatrick, F.J. (1988) *Ethics in Nursing Practice*, Linacre Centre, London.

Hargreaves, M. (1979) *Practical Law for Nurses*, Pitman Medical, Kent.

Jameton, A. (1984) *Nursing Practice: the Ethical Issues*, Prentice-Hall, Englewood Cliffs, NJ.

Murphy, C. and Hunter, H. (1983) *Ethical Problems in the Nurse–Patient Relationship*, Allyn, London.

NATN (1990) *Principles of Safe Practice in the Operating Department*, Harrogate, Yorks.

NATN, RCN and MDU (1988) *Theatre Safeguards*, London.

NBS (1985) 'Questioning of, or objecting to, participation in medical procedures', Guidance Paper, NBS, Edinburgh.

Pyne, R.E. (1981) *Professional Discipline in Nursing*, Blackwell, Oxford.

Quinn, C.A. and Smith, M. (1987) *Professional Commitment: Issues and Ethics in Nursing*, Baillière Tindall, London.

RCN (1977) *Ethics Related to Research in Nursing*, RCN, London.

Rumbold, G. (1986) *Ethics and Nursing Practice*, Ballière Tindall, London.

Sampson, A.C.M. (1982) *The Neglected Ethic: Religious and Cultural Factors in the Care of Patients*, McGraw-Hill, New York.

Speller, S.R. (1976) *Law Notes for Nurses*, RCN, London.

Tschudin, V. (1984) *Ethics in Nursing Practice*, Heinemann, London.

UKCC (1984) *Code of Professional Conduct for the Nurse, Midwife and Health Visitor*, UKCC, London.

Young, A.P. (1989) *Legal Problems in Nursing Practice*, Lippincott Nursing Series, Harper & Row, London.

7 The research process

RESEARCH METHODS

A knowledge of research methods is essential for nurses in the operating department for the following reasons:

- To enable the nurse to apply research findings in current practice.
- To conduct research and develop patient care.
- To audit existing practices and to set standards.
- To systematically collect data for management and theatre-utilisation data bases.
- To participate in multi-disciplinary research.

Until recently research was thought to be the prerogative of only a few nurses. With the advances in the health service and the move towards a quality service which is customer-led, knowledge about the research process and the application of research findings to practice are now central to contemporary nursing.

THE RESEARCH PROCESS

The research process, like the nursing process, can be broken down into component stages which are interrelated and sequential.

Defining the problem for investigation and searching the literature

This stage involves the identification of a problem for investigation. This is often more difficult than it first seems and involves consulting the literature on the topic of interest. Frequently, another researcher will have investigated the topic, and by searching the literature the nurse can learn of the methods used, the findings discovered and the implications of these findings to nursing. Sometimes it is just as valuable to replicate research conducted elsewhere, in order to determine if the findings are generalisable, as it is to design a new study.

At this stage it is also helpful to seek expert advice on research instruments and data analysis, and to discuss the ideas with other nurses, doctors and interested parties.

When searching the literature it is essential that the researcher keeps accurate records of the articles, books and papers consulted. This will be invaluable when it comes to writing the research report.

Planning the study

This is the stage when decisions are made about:

- The aims and objectives of the research.
- The methods to be used to investigate the problem.
- The time-scale and costs of the project.

The aims and objectives should be clearly stated and achievable and should relate directly to the problem under investigation. There should also be a correspondence between the objectives of the research and the methods used for investigation.

The methods used for investigation should include consideration of the sample of subjects who will be approached to participate, the rationale of the sampling techniques and the ethical aspects of the study. The research instruments which will be used to collect data must also be considered and possibly designed. The mode of analysis of the data should also be considered and also whether a pilot study requires to be conducted.

The time-scale of the project, from formulation of the problem to presentation of the research report, needs to be documented. This serves several purposes. Firstly, it enables the researcher to work to a timetable. Secondly, it ensures that time is allocated to each stage of the process. Thirdly, it ensures that those participating either directly or indirectly understand the timescale involved.

Methods of investigation

It is always advisable to conduct a pilot study. The results of the pilot study may reveal:

- problems in the design of the research.
- difficulties in obtaining access to the sample population.
- difficulties either in completing or in analysing the research instruments.
- problems with the time-scale of the project.

Collecting the data

There are many ways of collecting data. It is important to select the correct method or methods for the problem under investigation. Within the operating department the nurse may be asked to collect data as part of a clinical trial. Frequently, clinical trials are set up according to an *experimental design*. In the experimental design there is always at least one *experimental group* of subjects and one *control group* of subjects. The people in these groups are generally *randomly allocated*, and a particular product or drug is tested on the experimental group. The results obtained are then tested against the results of the control group, who will not have received the drug or the product under investigation. The researcher can then determine the efficacy of a particular product or drug.

Within nursing the research may be more exploratory or descriptive, and may involve some of the following methods.

Interview

When the data is collected by structured interview, the researcher has prepared a planned set of structured questions which will be put to all participants. The replies to the questions can be summarised and comparisons made.

The alternative interview technique involves asking unstructured questions. This method often yields rich data, as the answers to specific questions are elicited during free conversation. The distractions, omissions and disparities in replies that can and often do occur, however, make for difficulties in recording and interpretation.

Observation

There are two types of observation; participant and non-participant. In participant observation the researcher is part of the action, and is involved in and records events as they happen.

In non-participant observation the researcher observes actions without being directly involved. This is the method most frequently used in quality assurance techniques. Observation methods yield very rich data, but require considerable planning in advance in order to determine the framework and time-scale of the observations.

Questionnaires

Questionnaires that require written replies can be difficult to construct because of the necessity to avoid ambiguity and confusion. For this reason it is essential that all questionnaires are subjected to a pilot study.

Questionnaires, like interviews, can either be structured or unstructured. The structured questionnaire must have considered all the options and possible answers to questions, whereas the unstructured questionnaire enables the subjects to express themselves more freely. Structured questionnaires are easier to code and analyse than unstructured ones.

In designing any research instrument it is important to include the following:

- A brief explanation of the nature and aims of the study for the participants.
- A statement that all information gained will be treated confidentially and that respondents will remain anonymous.
- A statement of thanks to the participants for their cooperation and help.

ETHICAL CONSIDERATIONS

It is important to prepare an information sheet for subjects and to request their consent to participate in the research. Researchers have an obligation to respect the rights of individuals to refuse to participate in research without prejudicing their care or treatment. Individuals also have the right to withdraw from the project at any stage, again without fear of retribution.

If the research is sponsored commercially, the researcher must also consider any obligations to the sponsor and the effects of these on the ethics of the research.

For most research projects involving human subjects it is advisable to seek the advice and guidance of the Local Ethical Committee.

DATA ANALYSIS

The data collected requires to be sorted, coded and analysed. This may be carried out manually, and tables, graphs and diagrams produced. Alternatively, many nurses now have access to expert statisticians who will assist with the computerised analysis of data. Statistical packages are available which will produce descriptive, parametric and non-parametric statistics.

From the analysis of the data and knowledge of the literature the researcher can write the report and make recommendations for change or for further research.

WRITING THE REPORT

The research report usually follows the same logical sequence as that used to investigate the problem. It is important that the title reflects the problem under investigation. In constructing the research report, the following sections should be outlined:

1. Title page, with the author's name and qualifications.
2. Contents page.
3. Acknowledgements.
4. Research abstract or summary.
5. Introduction to the problem under investigation.
6. Review of the literature.
7. Method of investigation.
8. Data analysis.
9. Discussion of findings.
10. Conclusions, recommendations.
11. References and bibliography.
12. Appendices. These usually include the research instruments used in the study.

The nurse who is experienced and skilled in conducting research will be able to evaluate other research and determine which findings are the most valuable and should be implemented into nursing care.

Research is a specialised area of nursing with application in all clinical fields. Theatre nursing has the potential to be truly research-based. Although a wealth of pertinent research has been conducted in the United Kingdom and in North America, unfortunately many practices are still ritualistic and not founded on research. The challenge of the future is to make all nursing practice knowledge-based.

FURTHER READING

Ashworth, P. (1990) Bridges of opportunity: research linking nursing practice, education and management, RCN, Scutari, London.

Bergman, R. (1990) *Nursing Research for Nursing Practice: an International Perspective*, Chapman & Hall, London.

Berry, R. (1986) *How to Write a Research Paper*, Pergamon, Oxford.

Burnard, P. and Morrison, P. (1990) *Nursing Research in Action*, Macmillan, Basingstoke.

Burns, N. and Grove, S.K. (1987) *Practice of Nursing Research: Conduct Critique and Utilisation*, W.B. Saunders, Philadelphia.

Cormack, D.F.S. (ed.) (1990) *The Research Process in Nursing*, Blackwell, Oxford.

Fawcett, J. (1986) *Relationship of Theory and Research*, Appleton, Norwalk, CT.

Fitzgibbon, C. and Morris, L. (1987) *How to Analyse Data*, Sage, Newbury Park.

Hicks, C.M. (1990) *Research and Statistics: a Practical Guide for Nurses*, Prentice-Hall, Hemel Hempstead.

Hockey, L. and Macleod-Clark, J. (1979) *Research for Nursing*, HM&M Publishers, Aylesbury, Bucks.

Holm, K. and Llewllyn, J.G. (1986) *Nursing Research for Nursing Practice*, W.B. Saunders, Philadelphia.

Ogier, M. (1989) *Reading Research*, Scutari Press, London.

Pipkin, F.B. (1984) *Medical Statistics Made Easy*, Churchill Livingstone, Edinburgh.

Polit, D.F. and Hungler, B.P. (1987) *Nursing Research: Principles and Methods*, Lippincott, Philadelphia.

RCN (1977) *Ethics Related to Research in Nursing*, RCN, London.

Wilson-Barnett, J. and Robinson, S. (eds) (1989) *Directions in Nursing Research*, Scutari Press, London.
Woodward, M. and Francis, L. (1988) *Statistics for Health Management and Research*, Arnold, London.

8 The design and utilisation of the operating department

OPERATING DEPARTMENT DESIGN

Operating theatre design must meet the highest environmental criteria by providing optimum facilities whilst keeping expenditure as low as possible. Despite the fact that there has been an extensive building programme for hospitals in recent years, many operating departments are still a legacy of an earlier age. The physical environment no longer matches up to the remarkable modern achievements in surgery and the sophisticated equipment which is now in common use. The prime requirements in the design of a theatre are the control of infection and a safe and comfortable environment for the patients and staff.

The theatre complex should be located well away from other areas of the hospital and be completely self-contained. Designing the ideal operating theatre is a vast assignment, and the problems involved can only be solved by close cooperation between planners and engineers. Every step of the planning process presents the problem of either offering immediate facilities for today's developments or adapting to the new demands of further developments which are sure to come. The expertise of all theatre users must be considered and the knowledge of all the experts taken into account at each stage of planning. The findings of research into planning and design of operating theatres must be collected and analysed with the aim of providing a better basis for solving the problems faced by the planners.

All recommended proposals must conform to government standard requirements. Many theatres are now designed without windows, and here particular attention must be paid to correct lighting.

Certain essential points must be considered in the planning of an operating theatre complex:

1. Walls in the operating room must be finished in hard-wearing, easily cleanable material. Tiles or pannelled material should not be used because of the risk of cracks or falling plaster. Corners should be post-formed for maximum hygiene. Floors should be specially constructed to conduct electricity, should have a smooth finish for ease of cleaning, and should not have drains or gulleys.
2. There should be no ledges or shelves.
3. Facilities for piped oxygen, nitrous oxide, suction and scavenging devices should be incorporated in the design.
4. All electrical sockets and conduits must be earthed, and there must be an adequate number of them.
5. Fire-escapes, fire doors and equipment included in the building must conform to legal requirements.
6. An efficient and reliable air conditioning and heating system must be incorporated in the design.
7. Staff changing areas must be accessible from outside the theatre area.
8. A reliable emergency power supply must be available.

Overall design

In order to avoid cross-traffic and the risk of infection, the unit should be designed to allow entry at one side and exit at the other. Staff should have access to changing areas from outside, and patients can be admitted through a reception area for checking. If a holding area is incorporated in the design it should be located near to the reception area. Ideally two separate rooms should be allocated to care for adults and children. The rooms should be staffed by nurses, and the needs of both groups should be taken into account in decorating the rooms. Both should be sound-proofed and have subdued lighting. The children's area particularly should be appropriately decorated to lessen the fears of the child. It may be beneficial to have piped music in these areas.

Lounges, stock rooms, linen rooms and other ancillary rooms should be located on the outside of the theatre complex. They should be separated from the actual theatres by a dividing corridor.

There should be *direct* entry to the theatre from the anaesthetic room, and a hatch from the theatre should allow for the disposal of used equipment to a separate corridor for subsequent collection.

An area for preparation of equipment for surgery should be directly attached to the theatre, and the sinks for hand-washing should be adjacent. If pre-packed instrument sets are not used, a room must be incorporated in the design to allow for the cleaning and packing of sets.

Whether the design is for one operating theatre or a large complex, the most important consideration is to use the available space and money to best advantage. Careful planning should ensure that the actual theatre is completely separate from all other areas in the unit and that all patient traffic in the theatre leaves from a separate exit which leads to the recovery ward.

Recovery ward

The purpose of a recovery ward is to give total nursing care to the post-operative patient. Staff in this area must be particularly vigilant and have a sound knowledge of immediate post-anaesthetic and post-operative complications. Resuscitation equipment must be available and the room should incorporate facilities for piped oxygen and suction. General lighting should be efficient and there should be oxygen and suction available for each patient. Floors should be silent and easily cleanable, and doors should be wide enough to allow the passage of a bed and equipment. Temperature and ventilation control should be efficient, and an emergency power supply should be available. Hand-washing facilities are essential in this area, and so is a sluice room where bedpans, urinals and other essentials are stored. If possible, a partly partitioned area should be incorporated in the design. This can be used to nurse a particularly ill patient without causing unnecessary distress to other patients. If space permits, a section of the room can be used to nurse post-operative paediatric patients.

Anaesthetic room

Ideally, this room should be sound-proofed. It should be large enough to accommodate the patient's bed or trolley and the anaesthetic equipment and also allow sufficient space for staff to move freely. Whenever possible, equipment should be stored in cupboards: this will make the patient's experience far less frightening. A worktop should be available for the preparation of anaesthetic agents and other equipment. There is no reason why walls should not be pleasantly decorated, and the trend in recent years has been away from the more traditional lack of imagination in design where it was assumed that clinical white was essential. Floors in this room should be antistatic. Lockable wall cupboards should be available to accommodate scheduled and controlled drugs. Piped suction and oxygen, together with scavenging, should be incorporated in the room's design.

Steriliser room

If a Central Sterile Supply Department or Theatre Sterile Supply Unit (CSSD or TSSU) is impracticable, a room should be incorporated in the design to accommodate the sterilising equipment. However small the unit, this equipment should not be located within the actual theatre, as its use increases activity in the room and the increased heat and steam affect temperature control, increase humidity, adversely affect the performance of staff and increase the risk of infection. Particular attention should be paid to ventilation in the steriliser room.

Cylinder store-room

A high-ceilinged, well-ventilated, darkened room should be available to house the stock of cylinders.

Utility room

Each suite should have a room attached to it where cleaning equipment is stored. If a TSSU/CSSD is not in use, the room will need to be large enough to accommodate instrument trolleys where equipment can be washed and packed, but it is much safer to arrange that all instrument sets are packed in a separate room.

Reception area

This will be the first part of the theatre the patient will see, and it is vital that this first impression is of a pleasant and comforting place. As the reception area is not within the actual theatre, the risk of infection is less, so the design can be more ambitious. Cheerful colours can be used for walls, and pictures or wall plaques add a pleasant touch. The expense involved is minimal and the resultant benefit for the patient can be considerable. The area should be large enough to allow patients to be transferred from their bed or a trolley to the operating table or trolley, depending on local practice. Facilities such as desks and telephones for reception staff should be included here.

Theatre lighting

The range of activities within theatre suites requires better than average lighting. Any area in which the patient is cared for must have general lighting which is sufficiently bright to enable staff to detect any change in a patient's appearance or colour. These areas include corridors, anaesthetic rooms, theatre and recovery areas. Operating lights should provide cool, high-intensity illumination, with minimum glare.

ORGANISING THE DEPARTMENT

For an operating department to function effectively, good organisation is essential. In order to integrate a variety of skills, expertise, knowledge and technology in the interest of patients, care must be planned and the work of the department organised in terms of cost-effectiveness, quality of care and effective staffing.

Since the recent development of large operating departments, senior nursing staff have necessarily assumed responsibilities more far-reaching than the simple supervision of an operating session. During any one week issues may arise which test the staffing allocation to the full. For instance, if lists are allowed to run over-time on several occasions, staff with other responsibilities will be dissatisfied.

Several organisational goals for staff allocation have been specified in the literature and may be agreed on as follows:

1. The theatre timetable must be planned around the commitments of all grades of staff and professional responsibility and accountability towards patients.
2. A team leader should be assigned to each operating session to ensure the smooth running of the operating list.
3. Operating sessions must be planned to avoid peaks and troughs of activity and to allow essential maintenance to be carried out.
4. Time should be set aside purposely to allow members of the team to discuss any strategies and problems before surgery begins.

THE SIZE OF A THEATRE SUITE

Recommendations from various sources have stated that theatre suites allow for the concentration of operating facilities. This ensures maximum flexibility and economy of use in the programming of surgical work. The use of theatre suites also simplifies supply and disposal arrangements, and allows the maximum economy in staff, plant service rooms and running costs of the engineering services.

Furthermore, space economy is achieved by the centralisation of common ancillary accommodation (stores, staff-changing and rest rooms) and by the provision of recovery space as a single unit close to all theatres.

The optimum size for good organisation and staff morale has been identified as a complex of eight theatres. Such a size of theatre suite would satisfy the criteria identified above without causing too many staff-related problems.

ESTIMATING STAFFING

Established staffing formulas which have been devised for ward-based nursing and have nursing work-load per patient as their basis are not applicable in the operating department. In the operating department the nursing work-load is very high per patient for a short period of time. Furthermore, the nature of the work varies considerably in any one day, whereas in the ward situation the work-load remains fairly constant in terms of type of ward and number of beds.

Recommendations on theatre staffing levels and skill mix in the operating department have been set out by the National Association of Theatre Nurses, who suggest that a basic non-medical team of five persons should be available for each session, the leader of whom must be a qualified nurse. Furthermore, another member should be suitably trained to assist the anaesthetist and care for an unconscious patient.

NON-NURSING DUTIES

Non-nursing duties are often domestic or clerical in nature and are not related to nursing, but are essential to the smooth and effective running of an operating department. Research conducted by the present author has suggested that the employment of ancillary staff to ease the nursing work-load helps in the efficient running of the operating department. The necessary staff are as follows:

- Specific, designated portering staff to ensure the safe and speedy transfer of patients to and from the operating department.
- A well-trained and motivated domestic team to clean the operating department.
- A centralised instrument and sterile supplies service manned by designated staff.
- A secretary or receptionist within the operating department to undertake clerical and telephone duties.

FURTHER READING

Johnston, I.D.A. and Hunter, A.R. (eds) (1985) *The Design and Utilisation of Operating Theatres*, Arnold, London.

NATN (1987) *Quality Assurance Tool*, NATN, Harrogate.

NATN (1990) *Non-medical Skill-mix in the Operating Department*, NATN, Harrogate.

West, B.J.M. (1990) 'Managing an operating department', in *The Ward Sister's Survival Guide*, Austin Cornish, London.

9 Control of infection in the operating department

INTRODUCTION

Bacterial contamination continues to be the greatest hazard of surgery. All the diligence and skill of the surgical team will not produce the desired results unless every effort is made to avoid bacterial contamination of the surgical patient. Infection is the state or condition in which the body, or part of it, is invaded by pathogenic micro-organisms. Surgical sepsis results from many factors, one of which is bacterial contamination. Strict aseptic discipline must be applied at all times, and no amount of drugs, devices or architectural innovations can compensate for this. All staff in the theatre must cooperate in the application of recognised procedures, and managers must insist that they are adhered to.

Several factors may contribute to the rate and incidence of infection in the operating department. These include: the type of surgery performed, the skill of the surgeon, the patient's diagnosis and age, the length of stay in hospital, the duration of the procedure, host resistance, skin preparation, draping procedures, the number of organisms introduced into the wound during surgery, and environmental conditions in the theatre.

There are many activities involved in safeguarding the patient against infection:

- The adherence to established procedures in order to minimise the risks of infection by all staff.
- The adherence to a strict aseptic technique.
- The appropriate sterilisation of instruments, equipment, etc.
- Healthy, infection-free staff.
- A cleaning policy for the operating department.
- Adjustable and safe ventilation and humidity controls in each operating theatre.
- The adherence to guidelines on the movement and number of personnel involved during any surgical procedure.

For an infection to develop, three things must be present: infecting micro-organisms, a susceptible host and a method of transmission. Infection can be *endogenous*, in which the causative organism comes from another part of the patient's body, or *exogenous*, i.e. originating outside the body and acquired from another person or object. In the operating theatre, infecting micro-organisms can be reduced in numbers but not eliminated, hence the control of transmission is essential.

Operating theatres are comparatively free of organisms when empty, but the introduction of people immediately causes a sharp rise in the bacterial count. Opening and closing of theatre doors does not in itself increase the count, but a considerable increase is caused by the passage of people through the doors. In modern operating theatres the number of micro-organisms is reduced by cleaning and sterilising all equipment used. Staff wash their hands and forearms for a prescribed time before surgery to remove as many micro-organisms as possible, and they wear sterilised gowns and gloves.

The development of modern surgical techniques has been greatly advanced by an increased knowledge of the processes of the human body and the application of bacteriological research. Many operations which were previously considered dangerous because of the possible complication of infection can now be safely performed. This is partly due to the introduction of chemotherapy, especially prophylactic and therapeutic antibiotics.

THEATRE APPAREL

All persons entering the actual theatre must change into theatre clothing, and anti-static shoes should be worn. There has been continuous discussion over the years as to whether the wearing by female staff of trouser suits as opposed to dresses results in a lower release of organisms into the air. Results of research studies vary, but it seems that the general climate of opinion favours trouser suits. They are more practical, comfortable and flattering, and they reduce the desquamation rate. Cotton has been the material of choice for theatre clothes for many years, as it allows both circulation of air over the body and evaporation from the skin. There is no evidence to suggest that the wearing of loose-weave cotton clothing reduces contamination of the air by shed skin bacteria, but the use of Ventile, a close weave cotton, is shown to reduce considerably aerial dispersal of skin bacteria.

An operating theatre is, of necessity, an insular and often stressful area. The main consideration when selecting appropriate clothing must be patient safety, but it should be possible to design a uniform which is both safe and practical and also attractive in colour and design. This can only help in improving morale, and give staff the incentive to take a pride in their appearance. It will also help to make the patient's visit to the theatre less frightening. Far too many staff still wear ill-fitting, shapeless and often colorless garb in the mistaken belief that appearance is of little importance in an area which is so far removed from the rest of the hospital.

Tunic tops and tapered trousers should be available for male and female staff, with dresses for those who prefer them. White should be avoided: it does not improve with laundering and can also cause a certain amount of glare.

Footwear

A large range of comfortable theatre footwear is available on the market. Clogs, sandals, canvas shoes or wellingtons may be worn: all must conform to British standards for antistatic footwear. The use of overshoes is to be discouraged; despite considerable research, there is no evidence to suggest that wearing overshoes, either cotton or disposable, contributes in any way to a reduction in infection.

Masks

Exhalation of airborne bacteria from the nose and mouth is considered a prime source of pathogens, and generally masks are worn by all staff within the actual operating theatre. Manufacturers claim that disposable masks are effective for up to $2\frac{1}{2}$ hours. They are generally preferred to cotton masks, although some staff may be allergic to them. They should be fibre-free, lightweight and comfortable. When putting on a mask, it should be picked up by the tapes only, and tied securely ensuring that there are no loose ends. It should be changed at the end of a long operation and discarded on leaving the operating theatre.

Theatre headwear

All staff working within the actual theatre must ensure that their hair is completely covered. A wide range of attractive and practical headwear is now available in a variety of colours and designs. Where large numbers of staff are employed it may be useful to use different colours or patterns to denote grades. Disposable hats are popular because they are lightweight and comfortable to wear and they don't interfere with hearing. Helmet styles are also available for staff with longer hair.

SCRUBBING, GOWNING AND GLOVING

Powerful disinfection of the skin is impossible because of the damage a strong agent would cause, but all staff directly involved in a surgical procedure must spend a prescribed time rendering their hands as clean as possible. Individual hospitals will have their own policies, but there are certain basic principles that must be observed:

1. The first hand-wash of the day should last for five minutes or as long as it takes to ensure that hands are both socially clean and disinfected.
2. Disinfection should begin with cleaning, and ingrained dirt should be removed before the actual hand preparation begins.
3. Nails should be short and nail polish should not be worn.
4. Weak chemical agents can safely be used for hand-washing provided there is no skin cut or abrasion.

Agents in common use:

1. *Hexachlorophene* has a bacteriostatic action and its efficacy depends on regular and repeated use.

2. *Iodine-containing compounds* function by steadily releasing free iodine, and are non-staining.
3. *Ammonium compounds* are bactericidal and bacteriostatic. They are rapidly inactivated by any trace of soap left on the skin.

Procedure for handwashing

1. Turn on the water and ensure that it is warm and the flow moderate.
2. Wet and lather hands and arms with the selected agent.
3. Rinse off the lather and obtain a sterilized nail brush. This may be a re-usable brush or a pre-sterilized disposable one, which can be impregnated with a chemical agent.
4. Collect the agent from the dispenser on to the brush.
5. Holding the ends of the fingers and thumb evenly together, scrub the fingernails on one hand and repeat this procedure for the other hand.
6. Discard the brush by dropping it into the sink.
7. Rinse from fingertips to elbows.
8. Collect the agent in the palm of one hand.
9. Thoroughly wash the hands and arms, starting with the hands. Pay particular attention to the area between the fingers.
10. Finish wash at the elbows.
11. Rinse again from fingertips to elbows.
12. Hold the hands up and away from clothing.

PROCEDURE FOR DONNING STERILISED GOWN AND GLOVES

The gown will be prepared on a sterile towel by the circulator. Disposable hand towels can be included in the gown pack.

1. Pick up one towel so that it remains folded in half lengthwise.
2. Use one end of the towel to dry the hand, starting with the fingers.
3. Use the other end of the towel to dry the arm, using a slower circular motion. Never return to an area which has been dried.
4. Repeat the procedure for the other hand.
5. Discard the towel.
6. Pick up the gown firmly. It should be packed inside out to avoid the risk of touching the outside with the ungloved hand.
7. Find the top of the gown. (It is useful to have an indicator on gowns. This can be a coloured tab or a mark denoting the top.)
8. Hold the gown securely as it unfolds.
9. Bring the armholes into view and insert the arms.
10. Work both arms into the gown at the same time. (If the closed method of gloving is being used, push the hands to the inner edge of the cuff only. For the open method of gloving, push the hands through the cuffs.)
11. The circulator will tie the back tapes of the gown.

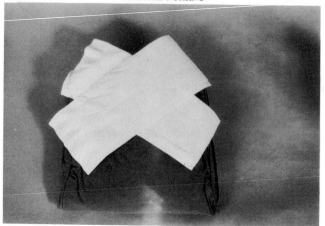

Figure 9.1 The gown pack is opened by the circulator.

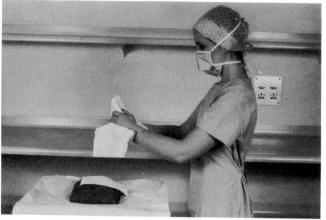

Figure 9.2 The nurse picks up the sterile towel and dries her hands, using one half for the hand and the other half for the arm.

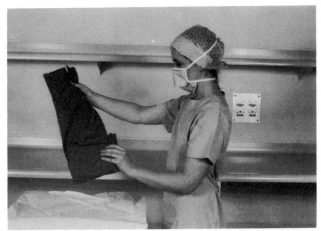

Figure 9.3 She then picks up the sterile gown and identifies the top.

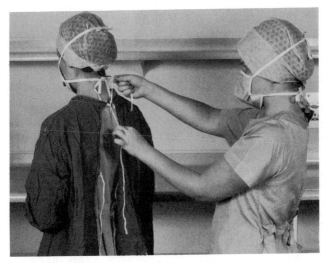

Figure 9.4 The circulator ties the back tapes of the gown.

Gloving

Closed method

The circulator will open the outer pack of the sterilised gloves.

1. With the thumb and forefinger collect the glove pack from inside the gown.
2. Put the pack on the sterile towel and open flat.
3. Through the gown, grasp the right glove with the left hand. Turn the right hand so that the palm is upward. Place the palm of the glove to the palm of the hand, with the thumb of the glove over the thumb of the hand.
4. Grasp the palm side of the glove cuff with thumb and forefinger, through the gown.
5. With the left hand, still inside the cuff, grasp the top cuff of the glove and pull it over the fingers.
6. Push the fingers into the glove. Grasp the sleeve and glove and pull on.
7. Repeat the procedure for the left hand.
8. Gloves can now be adjusted.

This technique is illustrated in Figures 9.5–9.9.

Open method

When the gown is put on, the hands are put through the cuffs (Figures 9.10–9.15).

1. The glove packet is collected from the circulator and placed flat on the sterile towel.
2. The packet of powder is removed from the glove pack and the hands are powdered. (This practice is not always used, as it is possible that the powder

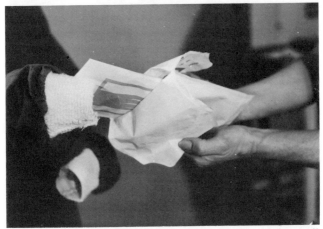

Figure 9.5 The circulator opens the outer packet of the sterile gloves.

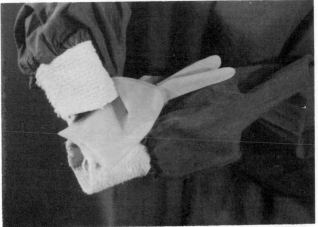

Figure 9.6 The palm of the glove is placed on the palm of the left hand and the glove cuff is grasped with the thumb and forefinger, through the gown.

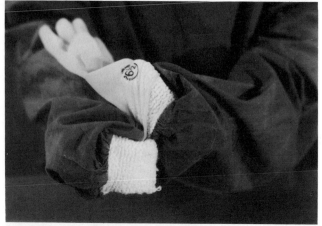

Figure 9.7 The glove is pulled over the cuff by the other hand, still inside the gown.

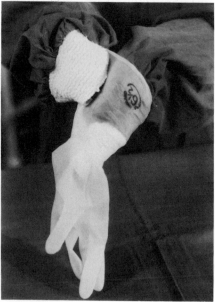

Figure 9.8

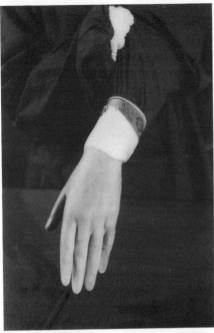

Figure 9.9 Adjust the glove by pulling up the sleeve.

could accumulate in a surgical wound, leading to the
formation of calculi.)
3. Pick up the left glove with the right hand, by the
   inside turned-down cuff.
4. Carefully push the fingers of the left hand into the
   glove until it reaches the cuff.
5. Pick up the right glove by putting the gloved hand
   under the cuff.
6. Carefully push the fingers of the right hand into the
   glove and pull the glove cuffs over the cuff of the gown.
7. Now pull the cuff on the left glove completely over
   the gown cuff of the left hand.
8. Adjust gloves.

This technique is illustrated in Figures 9.10–9.15.

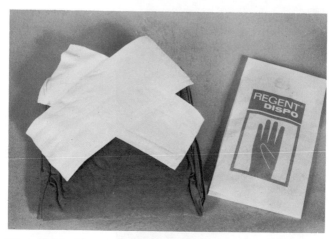

Figure 9.10 The gown pack and gloves are opened on a sterile towel by the circulator.

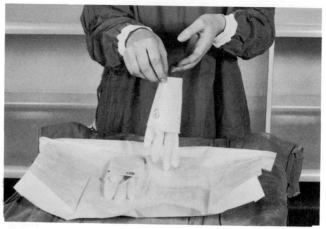

Figure 9.11 The glove packet is opened flat. The left glove is picked up by the right hand, touching the inside of the cuff only.

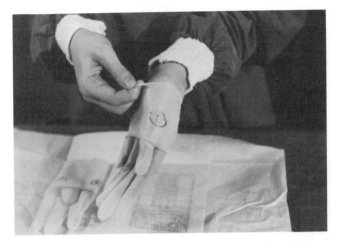

Figure 9.12   The hand is carefully inserted into the glove.

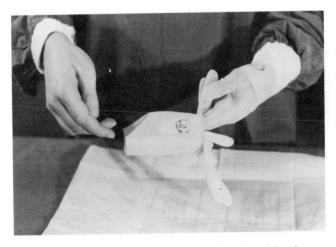

Figure 9.13   The procedure is repeated for the right glove.

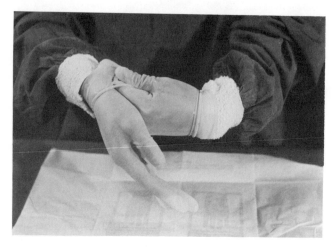

Figure 9.14   Both gloves are adjusted to cover the gown cuffs.

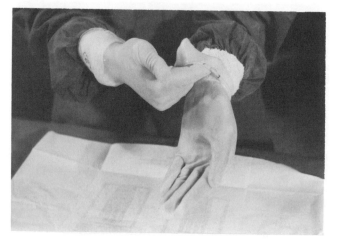

Figure 9.15

Plunge method

This method can only be used when one person is already gloved and gowned.

1. Pick up the glove with a gloved hand.
2. Insert the fingers of both hands under the cuff of the glove and hold it open.
3. Position the glove under the opened hand of the other person, glove thumb facing their thumb.
4. The other person now plunges his hand into the glove while the gloved person puts it completely over the gown cuff.

Adjusting gown

Surgical gowns must be designed to ensure that the back of the wearer is completely covered. The most commonly used type has a back panel which is folded over to the side before being sterilised. A tape from the panel is tied to a tape at the side of the gown. A removable tab of

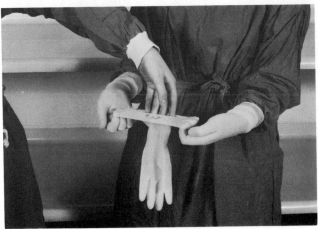

Figure 9.16 In the *plunge method* of gloving, the glove is held open and the hand is inserted.

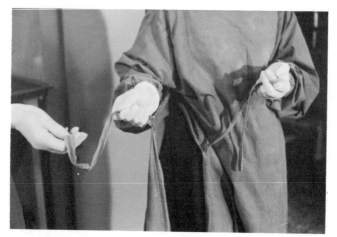

Figure 9.17 When gown and gloves are donned, the side tapes of the gown are untied and the tab is carefully handed to the circulator.

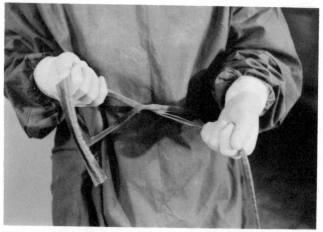

Figure 9.18 Both tapes are tied securely in front.

cardboard is attached to the panel tape when the gown is packed. When the gown and gloves are on, the tapes are undone and the tab (still attached) is handed to the circulator, who carefully rotates it around the gowned person. The circulator will then remove the tab, and both tapes can be tied.

Gloved hands should be held together and above waist level.

ASEPTIC TECHNIQUE

Principles of asepsis are always applied when carrying out any surgical procedure or any procedure which is likely to allow the entry of micro-organisms into the human body; e.g. insertion of central venous pressure lines, arterial lines, spinal or epidural anaesthetic cannulae or venesection.

The risk of introducing infection during any invasive technique must be minimised for the safety of the patient. The outcome of surgery depends on the creation and maintenance of an aseptic environment. Measures to prevent surgical wound infection include the provision of supplies and equipment which are free of microbial contamination at the time of use.

When participating in any aseptic technique it is important that the nurse is free of infected lesions of the skin or bacterial infections of the upper respiratory system. In addition, the nurse must ensure that the working environment and all trolley or other working surfaces have been thoroughly cleaned prior to the beginning of the operation. The packs and supplies to be used during the operation should be checked for sterility and date of expiry.

If the patient has an existing wound, then any dressings must be removed carefully from the wound in order to prevent scattering of micro-organisms into the air. This is usually carried out by the circulator, who wears gloves for protection. Because airborne cross-infection is a risk in the operating department, talking and movement within the operating theatre, opening and closing of theatre doors, exposing wounds and disturbing clothing and linen should be kept to a minimum.

STERILISATION AND DISINFECTION

There are no degrees of sterility. An object is either sterile or it is not. By sterility we mean that *all* micro-organisms have been killed.

Chemical disinfection differs from sterilisation in its ability to kill spores. Disinfection can be divided into three levels: high, medium and low. A high-level disinfectant can be sporicidal, bacteriocidal and virucidal if contact time is sufficient. A medium-level disinfectant is not sporicidal but will kill the more resistant bacteria and viruses. A low-level disnfectant will only kill the less resistant bacteria and viruses.

The length of time required to achieve sterilisation or high-level disinfection depends upon the following:

- The nature of the contaminating micro-organisms to be destroyed.
- The length of exposure to the sterilising or disinfecting agent required to produce the desired result.
- The bioburden of the object being sterilised or disinfected.
- The effective temperature required for the process to work.

Prior to sterilisation or disinfection all items should be thoroughly cleaned. The surrounding materials or packaging can interfere with the penetration of a sterilant. Therefore all packagings should be clean and conform to infection control standards.

Finally, when sterilising trays of instruments it is important that all surfaces are directly exposed to the sterilising agent for the prescribed duration and at the required temperature.

METHODS OF STERILISATION

Heat

Heat may be *dry* (hot-air ovens or infra-red conveyor ovens) or *moist* (steam).

Hot-air ovens

Ovens for sterilisation are electically heated and usually fitted with an internal fan to provide an even distribution of heat. Sterilising time is one hour at 160°C. This method is suitable for glassware, ophthalmic instruments and sealed tins or jars.

Infra-red conveyor ovens

Items are passed on a conveyor belt through a tunnel heated by infra-red elements. It is the effect of the heat and not the infra-red radiation which is lethal. Infra-red sterilisation is not commonly used nowadays.

Steam autoclaves

High-vacuum steam autoclaves are used to sterilise most equipment in common use, including dressings, metalware and instruments. Sterilising time is $3\frac{1}{2}$ minutes at a temperature of 134°C, with a total cycle time of approximately 40 minutes. This is the most widely used method of sterilisation, being economical and applicable to a wide range of items.

Low-temperature *steam-with-formaldehyde* autoclaves can be used to sterilise heat-labile materials such as 'scopes, plastics and anaesthetic equipment. Steam is admitted to a chamber under vacuum and formaldehyde is added: the vacuum keeps the steam temperature below 100°C. Without the addition of formaldehyde, only disinfection can be assured. Total sterilising and cycle times are variable, but are at least 2 hours at a temperature of 80°C. The disadvantages of steam/formaldehyde auto-claves are the long cycle time and the residual formal-dehyde, which is an irritant to living tissues.

Radiation

Ionising radiation, electron beams and gamma radiation are used on a commercial basis for the sterilisation of a wide variety of pre-packaged hospital articles. The items are exposed to a source of gamma rays, usually cobalt-60, within a thick-walled brick chamber. The total sterilising time is measured in days.

Gas

The sterilising gas (occasionally pure ethylene oxide but more usually 10–15 per cent ethylene oxide mixed with an inert gas, e.g. carbon dioxide) is pumped into a chamber containing the items for sterilisation. Total sterilising and cycle times, at 60°C and high humidities (over 70 per cent), are many hours.

This method can be used for a large range of heat-labile materials; e.g. implants, electrical apparatus, and anaesthetic machines and equipment.

CHEMICAL METHODS OF DISINFECTION

A wide range of chemicals are used as disinfectants. If they are to be effective, the manufacturer's instructions must be carefully followed.

The dangers associated with chemical disinfection are:

1. Many disinfectants gradually deteriorate after dilution with water.
2. If the same solution is used continually, its effectiveness will deteriorate.
3. There is always the risk of increased infection, because bacteria which survive in a disinfectant solution may multiply in it.

INSTRUMENT SETS

When pre-packed sets are used, instruments are prepared on a metal tray which is covered by a large drape that is secured to a rim on the tray. Swabs and drapes may also be included in this pack, depending on local policy. The drape is then folded over the tray and the set is double-wrapped in waterproof paper. Autoclave tape is applied and the set is lightly tied. The same principles are used when preparing metalware and drapes for sterilisation. This work is normally the responsibility of TSSU/CSSD staff, but nursing staff must also have adequate training in this department, as they may in some cases be responsible for the daily preparation of equipment. Instruments can be autoclaved in perforated metal tins which are wrapped in the same way as instrument sets.

Swabs, dressings and gloves are bought commercially and are disposable. All swabs used for surgery and anaesthesia must conform to the relevant British Standard and contain a radio-opaque marker.

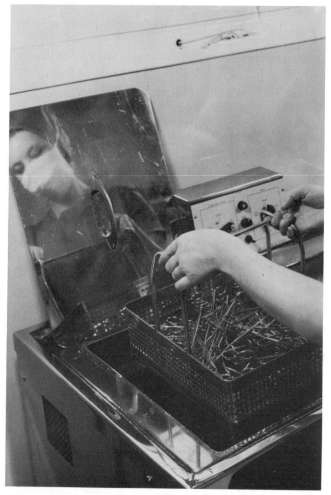

Figure 9.19 Instruments being washed in ultra-sonic washer (courtesy of Ultrasonics Ltd).

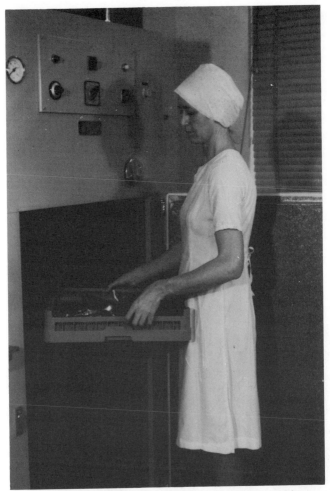

Figure 9.20 Instruments being placed in a drying cabinet.

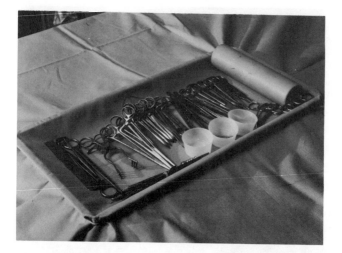

Figure 9.21 Instruments prepared on a covered tray.

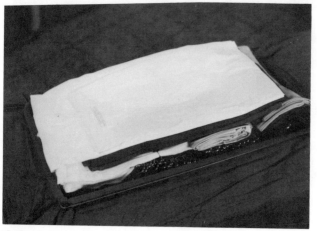

Figure 9.22 Swabs and drapes are added to the instrument set.

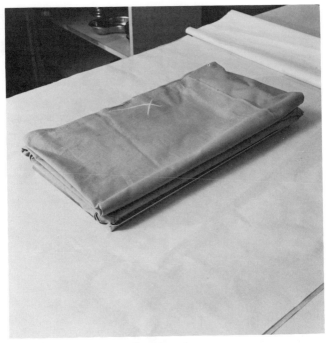

Figure 9.23 The draping towel is folded.

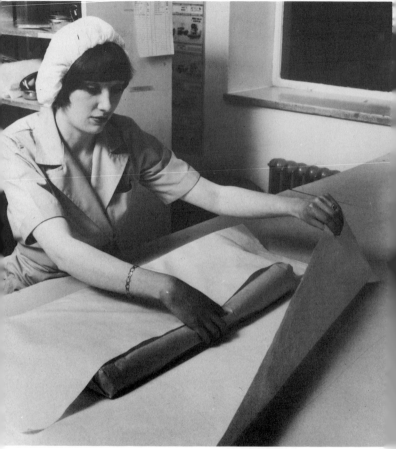

Figure 9.24   The set is double-wrapped in waterproof paper.

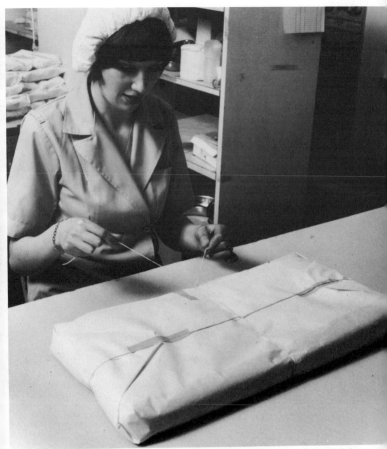

Figure 9.25 Autoclave tape is applied and the pack is lightly tied.

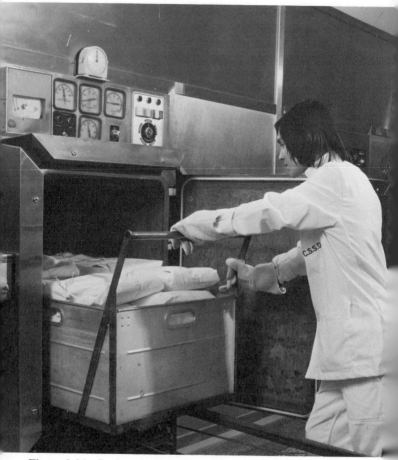

Figure 9.26   Packs are put into an autoclave for sterilisation.

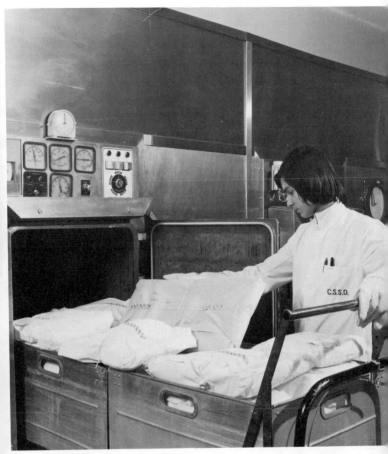

Figure 9.27 Sterilised packs are removed from autoclave.

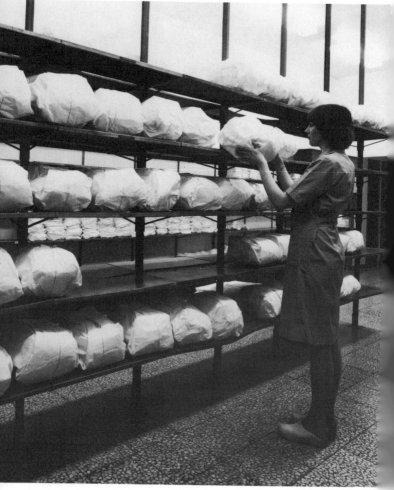

Figure 9.28 Sterilised packs are stored on shelves for delivery
to wards and theatres.

STERILISATION CONTROLS

1. *Spore test pieces* in common use are shown in Table 9.1. These offer a *guarantee* of sterility.
    Controls 2–7 merely indicate that certain conditions have been met, not necessarily that items are sterile.
2. *Chemical indicators* display colour changes. These may be brought about by changes in the temperature or pressure of gases, or by chemical changes due to radiation. Chemical indicators offer an immediate visual result.
3. *Browne's tubes* are small glass tubes partly filled with a red fluid which turns to green when a certain temperature has been maintained for a requisite period of time. Tubes are available to change at 120°C, 130°C, 160°C and 180°C.
4. *Diak tubes* are similar to Browne's tubes, except that a solid in the tube melts after the appropriate time at the required temperature.
5. *Autoclave tape* is a heat-sensitive tape which changes colour: a black stripe appears. A tape is also available

Table 9.1   Spore test pieces.

Process	Test spores	Test materials	Cultivation temperature
Moist heat (steam)	*Bacillus stearo-thermophilus*	Paper strips or discs	Broth at 55°C
Dry heat (hot air)	*Clostridium tetani*	Paper strips	Broth at 37°C
Ethylene oxide (gas)	*Bacillus globigii*	Foil strips	Broth at 37°C
Gamma radiation	*Bacillus pumilus*	Paper strips or discs	Broth at 37°C

All cultivation is aerobic, in broth, for 5 days.

for use with ethylene oxide gas: it is affected by the acid gas, whereupon a yellow stripe changes to red.

6. *Bowie and Dick test packs* are used for high prevacuum autoclave testing, in conjunction with various gauge readings, and give an indication of safe sterilisation. A sheet of paper on which there is a diagonal cross of autoclave tape is placed in the centre of a horizontal stack of approximately 29 folded huckaback towels. A uniform colour change throughout the tape within a period of $3\frac{1}{2}$ minutes at 134°C indicates safe sterilisation.

7. *Thermocouples* are used for testing heat methods of sterilising. Electrical leads with temperature-sensitive tips are placed in various parts of the sterilising chambers, and the leads passed through an aperture to a recording device outside. The temperature within the chamber can be constantly recorded throughout a cycle as a check that required temperatures are achieved and held for specified times.

CLEANING

The theatre should be cleaned at least one hour before the operating list commences. All flat surfaces, overhead lights and furniture should be damp-dusted with a disposable cloth, using fresh water to which a small amount of detergent has been added.

Floors must be cleaned whenever they are dirty, and if a particular theatre is not to be used during the night, the floor should be cleaned the previous evening.

Cotton mop-heads should be replaced after each use. The used head should be laundered and autoclaved before being used again. Sponge heads are also used and they must be treated in the same way. Ideally, floors should be cleaned by a machine which scrubs and suction-dries.

All other areas within the suite should be cleaned in the same way, and particular attention should be paid to the 'sluice' or disposal area. If mops are used for floor cleaning, the buckets should be kept in this area. They should be emptied and cleaned after each use and autoclaved regularly.

Cleaning between cases

Only areas which have become contaminated during the previous case should be cleaned.

Daily cleaning at the end of the day

The routine for daily cleaning is the same as that carried out before a list, but attention should also be paid to walls. Soiled areas should be cleaned with a disposable cloth.

Weekly cleaning

All furniture should be removed from the theatre and the floor should be washed. Ledges and permanent fixtures should be cleaned. Air-conditioning grills should be cleaned, usually by the contractor.

Contract cleaning of walls and ceilings

The frequency of wall- and ceiling-washing will be decided by the Control of Infection Committee. Some authorities maintain that this should be done weekly, but is is usually carried out every 3–6 months. A number of hospitals employ contract cleaners to undertake this task, in preference to direct labour.

Preparation of theatre for known status patients

If the cleaning policy is strictly adhered to, then no extra cleaning is necessary. All surgical patients deserve the same high standard of care in theatre, and modern philosophy suggests that provided these standards are maintained, it is not necessary or economical to institute a separate policy for known infected cases. The argument is that all surgery is a potential infection risk. Preparation of the theatre is the same as for other cases. Only essential equipment remains in the theatre and the number of personnel present should be kept to a minimum.

All staff should take precautions to avoid skin and mucous membrane contamination with *ANY PATIENT'S BLOOD OR BODY FLUIDS*.

Where the status of the patient is known then routine preparation should be as for all other cases, with the minimum of equipment in the theatre. Serum hepatitis and HIV are transmitted from person to person by inoculation of infected blood; e.g. from a contaminated suture or hypodermic needle. All mishaps during surgery should be reported immediately to the theatre manager and recorded in the patient's notes. Disposable drapes and equipment should be used, and all staff involved in the case should wear protective gowns and gloves.

ALL disposable material should be placed in yellow bags (double-bagged), sealed and labelled with 'Bio-hazard' notices.

Sharps used must be placed in a non-permeable container and labelled with Biohazard tape. Any linen used should be placed in special bags, sealed, then placed in laundry bags which have been labelled for infected wash procedures.

Instruments should not be hand-washed but bagged, labelled and sent for treatment. Finally, it is imperative to avoid contamination with any blood or body fluids.

FURTHER READING

Block, S.S. (1983) *Disinfection, Sterilisation and Preservation* (3rd edn), Lea & Febiger, Philadelphia.

Brigden, R. (1989) *Operating Theatre Technique*, Churchill Livingstone, Edinburgh.

British Standard (1981) *Guide to Good Manufacturing Practice*, BS 5750.

Institute of Sterile Service Managers (1989) 'Guide to good manufacturing practice' (Dec.).

NATN, *Principles of Safe Practice in the Operating Theatre – a Resource Book*, NATN, Harrogate.

Perkins, J.J. (1983) *Principles and Methods of Sterilisation in Health Sciences*, Charles Thomas, Springfield, IL.

10   Surgical instrumentation

Special instruments have been crafted for specific operations, and the inexperienced nurse may feel daunted by the range of surgical instruments available. All surgical instruments are made precisely and must conform to specific standards and specifications.

Usually a stainless steel alloy is chosen for manufacturing the instruments as this is not susceptible to rust. Frequently, tungsten carbide is incorporated to reinforce particular parts of the instruments, and those instruments which will be used in electro-surgery will always be insulated.

CRITERIA FOR NAMING INSTRUMENTS

Surgical instruments are generally named by the use to which they are put; e.g. an artery forcep; a dissecting forcep; a tissue forcep; a bowel clamp. In addition, the name of the designer is often added; so, for instance, a Dunhill artery forceps; a McIndoe dissecting forceps; a Babcock tissue forceps and a Peyrs bowel clamp. A further classification is often added, and that is the length or size of the instrument; e.g. a 7-in. Babcock tissue forceps.

CLASSIFICATION OF INSTRUMENTS

Surgical instruments can be classified into six basic groups. These are:

- Cutting and dissecting instruments.
- Grasping or holding instruments.
- Clamping instruments.
- Exposing instruments.
- Investigating instruments.
- Suturing instruments.
- Sponge-holding instruments.

A basic instrument set for all types of surgery will comprise an assortment of the above types of instruments (Fig. 10.1, p. 184). The following list is given as an example:

Sponge holders

(Long and short lengths)

Knife handles × *3*

(for large and small blades)

Dissecting forceps

(Toothed and non-toothed, 5 and 7 ins in length)

Scissors

(Straight-bladed and curved-bladed, various lengths)

Artery forceps

(Curved and straight of various lengths)

Tissue-holding forceps

(Heavy and light)

Needleholders

(Various lengths)

Retractors

(With various depths of blades, hand-held and self-retaining)

Diathermy instruments and quiver

In addition, specialist equipment will also be added to the set in surgical specialities. Each set will have a contents list against which the scrubbed assistant and the circulator will check the contents. (Examples of instruments in common usage are shown in Figures 10.2 to 10.7, pp. 185–188).

HANDLING SURGICAL INSTRUMENTS

It is important that the nurse touches the handles of instruments rather than the operative ends in order to minimise the risk of contamination.

When passing instruments during an operation, the aim is to pass the instrument into the surgeon's hand ready for use. This requires an awareness of ergonomics and knowledge of how the instrument will be used. When passing artery forceps, tissue forceps or scissors it is best to hold them in the middle and place the handle of the instrument in the surgeon's palm. If the instrument is curved, then the curve most frequently points inwards.

When passing dissecting forceps, hold them at the lower ends in order that the surgeon can grasp the top end and use them immediately. Retractors should be passed so that the surgeon receives the blades to position in the wound.

Passing the scalpel requires care in order that no injury occurs to the patient, the nurse or the surgeon. The nurse should hold the scalpel handle towards the blade end from above, with the cutting edge of the blade facing downwards and the handle end pointing slightly upwards. This enables the surgeon to grasp the scalpel handle, and the cutting edge of the blade is drawn away from the nurse.

GENERAL AND MINOR SETS

The use of pre-packed instrument sets has simplified the preparation of instruments for surgery. Whether the sets are supplied from a Central Sterile Supply Department (CSSD) or prepared by staff in the theatre, it is both useful and time-saving to have basic sets to which particular instruments can be added for extensive procedures. The disadvantage of acquiring a large number of basic sets is the initial financial outlay, but this is more than compensated for in the saving of nursing time and in the fact that lists are not held up waiting for instruments to be sterilized between cases.

For ease of identification, sets can be classified as General or Minor sets. A General set can be used for most operations on the abdomen, with the addition of some special instruments for particular operations. A Minor set can be used for less extensive surgery; e.g. hernia repair or excision of a lump in the breast. The contents of a General set are given in Fig. 10.1. These instruments may be used in a general surgical theatre. However it should be remembered that the instruments used vary according to local practice and the surgeon's preference.

POWER TOOLS

Within many surgical specialities power tools are used. These can be either electrically or pneumatically driven instruments, and are used for drilling or sawing. The advantages of such tools are that they cause less trauma and pain to surrounding tissues and are more precise than hand-operated saws or drills.

Many of these tools are composed of a power driver and interchangeable attachments, such as drilling chucks and saw blades. Prior to use, each of the attachments must be tested to ensure correct assemblage. The power driver must not be immersed in water but can be gas- or steam-autoclaved.

ENDOSCOPES

In the last decade there has been a tremendous advance-ment in the production of endoscopic equipment. These instruments are invaluable aids to diagnosis and to the execution of surgical procedures.

Rigid endoscopes are available, and are used for:

- Laparoscopy.
- Thoracoscopy.
- Laryngoscopy.
- Oesophagoscopy.

Flexible fibre-optic endoscopes (Figures 10.8 and 10.9, p. 189 and p. 190) are now available for:

- Bronchoscopy.
- Oesophagoscopy/Gastroscopy.
- Colonoscopy.
- Duodenoscopy.

Each of these endoscopes, whether rigid or flexible, can be used to perform surgery. Within the last five years laparoscopic abdominal surgery has been pioneered using either diathermy or laser via a laparoscope for excision and coagulation.

Laparoscopic cholecystectomy is now performed regularly throughout the United Kingdom. Such advances in surgical technique will continue to make the patient's stay in hospital shorter and recovery quicker.

CARE OF SURGICAL INSTRUMENTS

All surgical instruments should be tested and inspected prior to and after use in order to minimise any risk to the life of the patient. When inspecting surgical instruments it is essential that the nurse checks that:

- All the component parts of the instrument are present and in good working order.
- The joints of instruments are free from obstruction and operate smoothly.
- The ratchet fastenings of instruments grip firmly in each setting.
- The points of dissecting forceps are in alignment.
- The scissors are sharp.
- The diathermy instruments are insulated.
- Cannulated instruments are free of obstruction.

CLEANING SURGICAL INSTRUMENTS

In many hospitals this will be carried out by designated staff working in theatre sterile supplies units. When any member of staff is involved in cleaning a surgical instrument, it is imperative that the individual adheres to the universal precautions regarding blood and body fluids.

The instruments are usually washed in a special detergent, rinsed, dried and then sterilised. The washing may be carried out by hand or in specially designed washing machines.

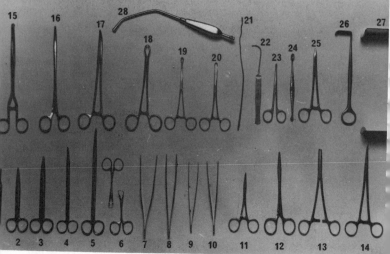

Figure 10.1 General set.

1. Bard Parker handle × 2
2. Mayo's curved scissors
3. Mayo's straight scissors × 2
4. McIndoe's dissecting scissors
5. Nelson's dissecting scissors
6. Towel clips × 8
7. Toothed dissecting forceps
8. Non-toothed dissecting forceps
9. Gillie's dissecting forceps
10. McIndoe's dissecting forceps
11. Dunhill artery forceps × 10
12. Spencer Well's artery forceps × 10
13. Oschner artery forceps × 4
14. Lahey artery forceps × 4
15. Sponge holder × 4
16. Roberts artery forceps × 2
17. Moynighan artery forceps × 2
18. Lane's tissue forceps × 2
19. Babcock tissue forceps × 2
20. Allis tissue forceps × 2
21. Probe
22. Aneurysm needle
23. Sinus forceps
24. Volkman's spoon
25. Mayo's needle holder × 2
26. Langenbeck retractor × 2
27. Morris retractor × 2
28. Pharyngeal sucker

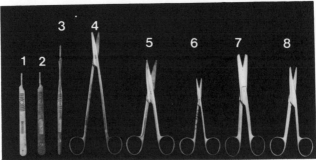

Figure 10.2 A selection of scalpels and scissors.
1. No. 4 Bard Parker handle: used with No. 21, 22, 23, 24 and 25 blades
2. No. 3 Bard Parker handle: used with No. 10, 11, 12 and 15 blades
3. No. 7 Bard Parker handle: used with No. 10, 11, and 15 blades
4. Nelson's lobectomy scissors
5. Large curved Mayo's scissors
6. Fine curved plastic scissors
7. Large straight Mayo's scissors
8. Small curved Mayo's scissors

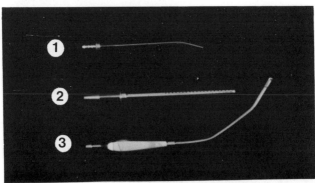

Figure 10.3 Suction nozzles.
1. McIndoes
2. Sump
3. Yankauer

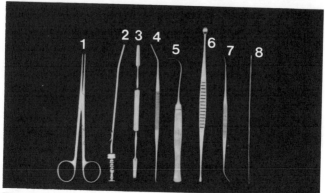

Figure 10.4 Additional instruments for use with basic sets.

1. Sinus forceps
2. Gillie's fine suction nozzle
3. McDonald's double-ended dissector
4. Gwen-Evan's double-ended dissector
5. Aneurysm needle
6. Large Heath double-ended spoon
7. Watson Cheyne's probe dissector
8. Single-ended probe

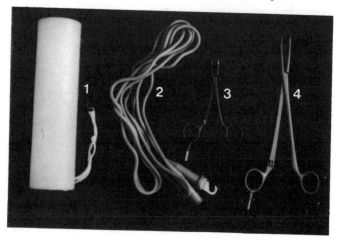

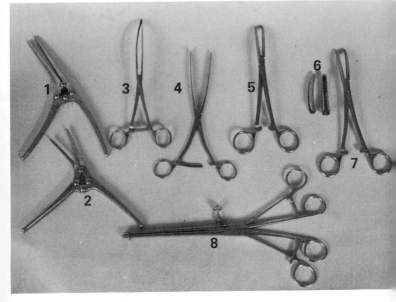

Figure 10.6 A selection of intestinal clamps.

1. Payr crushing clamp, small
2. Payr crushing clamp, medium
3. Doyen occlusion clamp, curved
4. Doyen occlusion clamp, straight
5. Joll crushing clamp
6&7. Parker-Kerr crushing clamp with guard
8. Lane's twin occlusion clamp

Figure 10.5 (facing page)   Diathermy for use with basic sets.

1. Quiver
2. Lead
3. Small Riche's forceps
4. Large Riche's forceps

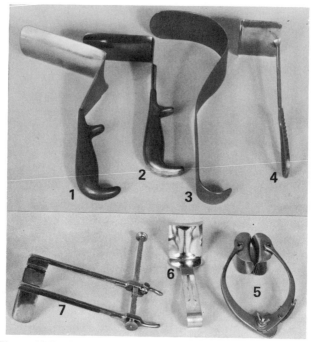

Figure 10.7 Retractors in common use

1. St. Mark's
2. Liver
3. Deaver
4. Morris
5. Ricard Begonin
6. Middle blade for Ricard Begonin
7. Gosset's

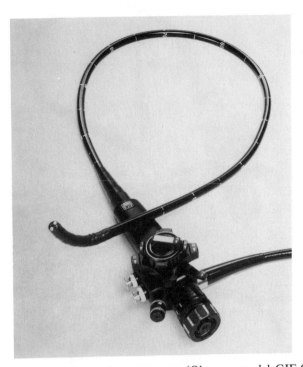

Figure 10.8 Fibreoptic gastroscope (Olympus model GIF-Q). This is an example of one of the many types of fibre-optic gastroscopes currently in use. The use of this flexible endoscope allows for examination of the oesophagus, stomach or duodenum. Diathermy forceps are also available and the instrument is designed for the attachment of a camera.

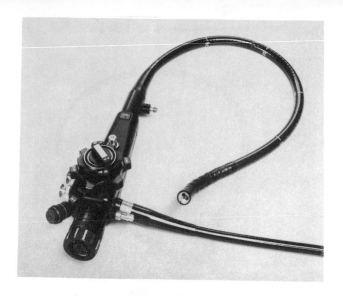

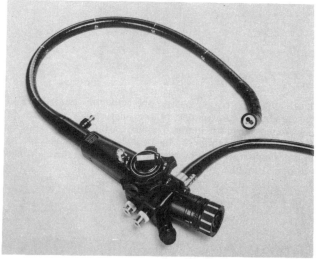

Figure 10.9 Flexible sigmoidoscopes. These are examples of one type of flexible sigmoidoscope. Flexible, fibre-optic colonoscopes are also available.

FURTHER READING

AORN (1988) 'Care of instruments, scopes and powered surgical instruments', *Journal of American Operating Room Nurses*, 47(2).
NATN, *Principles of Safe Practice in the Operating Department – a Resource Book*, NATN, Harrogate.

11 Wound healing and sutures

WOUND HEALING

A large variety of materials can be used for closure of incisions, ranging from synthetic fibres to staples and adhesive strips. The surgeon will use the material which is best suited to the particular operation, taking into account the healing properties of the patient, whether or not the wound is already infected, the particular disease, and his past experience of different suture or stapling materials.

The purpose of suturing or stapling is simply to hold the wound together until it heals through the natural healing process. The immediate strength of a wound is dependent on its sutures or staples, and if healing is delayed for any reason, continued support may be necessary.

Various factors determine the time it takes for a suture or staple line to heal, including:

1. The suturing skill of the surgeon and the gentleness with which he handles tissue.
2. The type of tissue and the site of suturing (e.g. cardio-vascular surgery is a special case).
3. The physical condition of the patient. Healing is likely to be rapid in a young, healthy patient, whereas conditions such as anaemia, diabetes, obesity, cancer and malnutrition can delay healing and predispose to wound infection.

4. Existing sepsis.
5. Decreased oxygen tension.
6. Recent radiation therapy.
7. Some drug therapy; e.g. cortisone, immunosuppress-ive drugs.
8. The presence of a foreign body; e.g. a swab or instrument, in the wound.
9. Insertion of a drain in the suture line.
10. Inefficient aseptic technique.
11. Ineffective sterilising methods.
12. Wound closure.

The process of surgical wound healing involves distinc-tive stages. With surgical wounds the intention is to encourage healing by primary union. This occurs in clean incised wounds where there has been little or no loss of tissue and the wound edges are in close opposition. The space between the two cut surfaces fills with plasma, which forms a sticky medium into which fibroblasts and vascular endothelial cells grow. This usually occurs within the first 24 hours. At the same time the endothelial lining of the capillaries proliferates and forms a branching network. The narrow gap is bridged by endothelial cells, which grow in from the wound edges.

The process of inflammation

This can be defined as the response of the body to an irritant and involves four distinctive stages. These can be classified as follows:

1. Traumatic inflammation

During this stage the edges of the wound become oedematous and are matted together with fibrin. The capillaries dilate, and fluid collects in the interstitial space and may leak through the damaged endothelium.

2. Destruction phase

During this phase all necrotic tissue is removed by the migration of leucocytes and macrophages into the wound. These special cells engulf and destroy dying tissue.

3. Proliferation phase

This is the stage when the epithelium and connective tissues develop new capillaries and fibroblasts appear. These two structures together comprise granulation tissue. This stage usually starts between day 4 and day 14. During this stage all the cells which make up the surface epithelium undergo rapid division and migrate, thereby producing a thin film which covers the wound.

4. Maturation phase

At this stage blood vessels gradually disappear and the number of fibroblasts in relation to fibres diminishes. The red elevated scar soon diminishes into a white line.

Healing by granulation

This occurs when there is loss of tissue or infection present. Because the fibroblasts are incapable to joining the wound surfaces together, repair starts at the base of the wound. The wound defect becomes filled with blood clot, plasma and inflammatory exudate. The resultant granulation tissue is highly vascular and is composed of fibroblasts, vascular endothelial cells and morphonuclear leucocytes which ingest bacteria and keep the wound free from serious infection.

Bone healing

This involves the formation of osteoid tissue, the deposition of calcium and phosphorus.

Granulation tissue forms in the haematoma which surrounds the bone ends. The fibrous tissues formed differentiate into fibrocartilage. Almost simultaneously osteoblasts proliferate and a loose callus forms a sleeve around the fracture ends. This tissue unites and helps to stabilise the fracture. Gradually more calcium and phosphorous salts are deposited in order that true bone can be formed. Tissues are then restructured and remodelled.

Factors affecting wound healing

1. *Poor arterial blood supply. This may be due to:*

   - Arteriosclerosis.
   - Cardiogenic shock.
   - Arterial thrombus.
   - Prolonged use of a tourniquet.
   - Tight, restrictive wound dressings.

2. *Deficient venous drainage. This may be due to:*

   - A deep vein thrombosis.
   - Varicose veins.

3. *Deficiency or depression of blood. This may be due to:*

   - Anaemia.
   - Leucopenia.
   - Hypoproteinaemia.

4. Poor nutritional state or malnutrition.
5. Dehydration.
6. Metabolic disorders.
7. Certain drug therapies; e.g. cortico-steroids.

SUTURES

Gauge

Sutures and ligatures come in various diameters and
tensile strengths. Table 11.1 shows the range of suture
materials currently available.

The metric gauging system of suture materials has now
been adopted by both the European and the US
pharmacopoeias. The metric number represents the
diameter of the suture in tenths of a millimetre. Equivalent
gauges are shown in Table 11.2.

NEEDLES

Needles used for surgical suturing vary according to
heaviness, length, the shape of the needle and the point
of the needle. The heaviness of the needle will correlate
with the gauge of the suture, thereby producing an
atraumatic suture (Fig. 11.1). So, generally speaking, the
thicker the suture, the greater the tensile strength and
the thicker the needle.

The length of the needle will depend upon the thickness
of the tissue to be sutured. The shape of the needle will
depend upon access to the tissue to be sutured and the
wish to cause minimal trauma to surrounding tissues.

Needle points are more differentiated. They fall into
two broad categories:

- Needles with a *cutting edge*. These are used to suture
  tough tissue.
- Needles with a *round body*. These are used to suture
  more delicate and friable tissue.

Figure 11.2 demonstrates the range of needle points
available.

Table 11.2 Metric gauging of suture material.

Metric gauge Metric number	Catgut/collagen	Former gauge Non-absorbables and synthetic absorbables
0.1	–	–
0.2	–	10/0
0.3	–	9/0
0.3	–	8/0 virgin silk
0.4	–	8/0
0.5	8/0	7/0
0.7	7/0	6/0
1	6/0	5/0
1.5	5/0	4/0
2	4/0	3/0
3	3/0	2/0
3.5	2/0	0
4	0	1
5	1	2
6	2	3&4
7	3	5
8	4	6

Reproduced by kind permission of Ethicon (Edinburgh).

STAPLING TECHNIQUES

Stapling devices are available for:

- Skin closure.
- Performing entero-entero anastamoses.
- Performing transverse anastamoses.
- Dissecting and anastamosing simultaneously.
- Ligating blood vessels.

These products have greatly reduced the duration of operations and therefore the length of time a patient is subjected to an anaesthetic.

Table 11.1 Suture materials in common use.

Suture	Types	Source	Absorption	Some uses
Surgical gut	Plain	Collagen from animals	Absorbed quickly, by enzyme action	Ligation of superficial blood vessels; suturing of subcutaneous tissues
Surgical gut	Chromic	Collagen treated with chromium salts	Absorbed more slowly, by enzyme action	Fascia; peritoneum. Versatile suture and ligature
Vicryl	Braided	Copolymer of lactide and glycolide	Absorbed by hydrolysis slowly	Ligature or suture where absorbable material suitable
PDS	Mono-filament	Copolymer of polydiaxanone	Absorbed by hydrolysis slowly	Versatile suture
Dexon	Braid	Polymer of galactin and lactide	Absorbed by hydrolysis	Versatile suture and ligature

Name	Type	Material	Absorption	Uses
Prolene	Mono-filament	Polymer of propylene	Non-absorbable	Versatile suture. Fine gauge used in vascular surgery
Nurolon	Braided	Polyamide Polymer	Non-absorbable	Versatile suture and ligature
Ethilon	Mono-filament	Polyamide Polymer	Non-absorbable	Muscle, skin and for tension suturing
Ethibond	Braided	Polyester	Non-absorbable	Strong wound closure; tendon repair
Surgical silk	Braided	Natural protein	Non-absorbable	Versatile suture and ligature (rarely used)
Surgical cotton	Twisted	Natural cotton	Non-absorbable	Versatile ligature (rarely used)
Surgical steel	Mono or multi	Alloy of iron	Non-absorbable	Rarely used

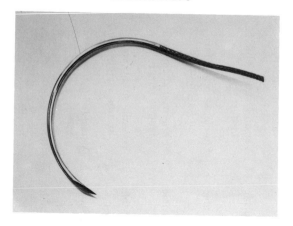

Figure 11.1 Atraumatic suture.

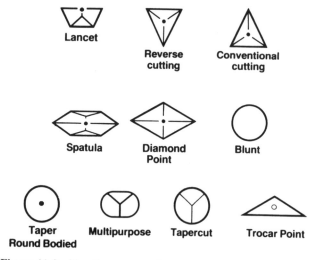

Figure 11.2 Needle cross-sections.

FURTHER READING

Brigden, R. (1989) *Operating Theatre Technique*, Churchill Livingstone, London.

NATN (1991) *Principles of Safe Practice in the Operating Department: A Resource Book,* NATN, Harrogate.

12 Hazards in the operating department

INTRODUCTION

The avoidance of accidents to patients and staff is of paramount importance in this area, and legislation highlights the responsibility of theatre managers to ensure a safe environment. The Health and Safety at Work Act 1974 clearly states that 'every employer has a duty to ensure the health, safety and welfare at work of all his employees so far as is reasonably possible' and that 'every employee has a duty while at work to take reasonable care for the health and safety of himself and of other persons who may be affected by his acts or omissions at work'.

The increasing use of new and sophisticated equipment can increase the risk of accidents. Theatre staff must have instruction in the use of all new equipment, and manufacturers are generally very willing to assist in this teaching.

The role of the theatre nurse is continually developing as changes in practice add new dimensions to the range of nursing duties. The performance of these duties may well mean that the nurse is functioning in an extended role for which there has been no training and which is not legally covered. Under civil law procedures, *individual* responsibility can be placed on a nurse, and it is essential that employing authorities issue contracts which fully cover the range of duties of an employee and define their operational policy relating to indemnity insurance requirements.

Effective management and a policy of continuing education for all staff should help to prevent many of the possible hazards in the theatre.

Faulty design

Many theatres are a legacy of a bygone age, but because of financial constraints they continue to be used. In many cases drains and gulleys provide a breeding ground for bacteria, windows are the only form of ventilation, instruments are boiled within the theatre, and doors open directly on to main hospital corridors. Despite these handicaps, the infection rate in such theatres may still be low, and this can only be attributed to the skill of the theatre staff.

Pollution from anaesthetic gases

There is a continuing need to inform staff of the pollution hazards in the theatre, and in compliance with the Health and Safety at Work Act suitable anaesthetic gas scavenging systems should be fitted.

Unsatisfactory methods of sharps disposal

A large number of 'sharps', e.g. blades and needles, are used in operating theatres, and their disposal can create a very serious hazard. A good disposal system will protect not only theatre staff but also porters and laundry workers. Such 'sharps' must be discarded immediately after use and an appropriate sealed container should be available wherever they are used, whether in the anaesthetic room, recovery ward or theatre.

Absence of safety signs

A uniform system of safety signs and colours for use throughout the EC came into effect in January 1981. These signs are intended to give health and safety messages by use of a combination of geometrical shapes, colours and pictorial symbols. There are prohibitive, caution and hazard signs. Full details of the signs are given in the Health and Safety Commission/British Standards Institution Statutory Instrument No. 1471.

Other avoidable hazards in theatre

These include non-adherence to agreed policies on:

1. Fire prevention.
2. Sterilisation methods.
3. Cleaning procedures.
4. Aseptic technique.
5. Patient identification procedures.
6. Swabs, needles and instrument count.
7. Disposal of used material.
8. Record keeping.
9. Patient safety.

Many of these hazards can be avoided if staff are kept informed of new developments and legislation and multi-disciplinary standards are developed.

RADIATION

Ionizing radiation can be obtained from X-ray machines, high-energy accelerators, nuclear reactors or radioactive isotopes. Artificial radioactive isotopes can be used as radiation sources, the most widely used being cobalt-60 and caesium-137.

Diagnostic radiography

The current unit of X-ray exposure is the roentgen, and the unit of absorbed dose is the rad. These will be replaced by new units consistent with the International System of Units (SI), in which the unit of absorbed dose is the Gray (symbol Gy) = 1 joule per kg, and the unit of exposure is 1 coulomb per kg. No special name has been assigned to the unit of exposure, which is approximately 3876 roentgens.

Radiography has become a necessary adjunct to surgery, and adequate protection must be provided for staff in the theatre. X-radiation, like all electro-magnetic and ionising radiation, follows the inverse square law: if at 1 metre away you receive x units of radiation, when you move 2 metres away you receive only $x/4$ units, at 5 metres only $x/25$ and at 10 metres only $x/100$.

Safety precautions when using X-ray equipment

1. Wall switches should be of the enclosed mercury type to prevent any possibility of sparking.
2. The X-ray beam should be confined to as small an area as possible.
3. Only staff directly involved in the procedure should remain in the theatre.
4. Staff should wear lead-rubber aprons which have a minimum lead-equivalent of 0.25 mm for X-rays excited at voltages up to 150 kV: protective gloves, with the same lead-equivalent, should be worn if the hands are likely to be close to the beam.
5. Theatre staff who are likely to receive a significant dose of X-radiation must be provided with a film badge or pocket dosimeter.
6. Female staff-members who are pregnant should be advised NOT to participate in X-ray procedures.

Radiotherapy implants

Theatre nurses will encounter most radiation hazards when dealing with patients who are receiving treatment with radioactive sources, such as those illustrated in Table 12.1.

Table 12.1

	Half-life
radium	1,620 years
caesium-137	33 years
cobalt-60	5.3 years
iridium-192	74 days
grains of gold-198	2.7 days
yttrium-190	2.54 days

These sources may be inserted in the theatre as intracavity sources, e.g. within the cervix, or the applicators may be inserted and the sources loaded on return to the ward.

Intracavity sources

The use of radium tubes in the treatment of carcinoma of the cervix is being superseded by caesium tubes of like dimensions and activities. When radium is the treatment of choice, the sources are inserted under general anaesthetic and secured with packing. A self-retaining catheter is also inserted to facilitate post-operative nursing care.

1. The most effective protection for all staff is distance combined with speed of operation, although heavy lead shielding is also used. In this connection it should be emphasised that lead rubber aprons afford

no protection from the radiation emitted by sources other than mobile X-ray units, and they are an unnecessary and useless encumbrance during intracavity and interstitial procedures.

2. The sources should be contained in a lead pot, and this must be transported from the main store to the theatre in a container which provides adequate protection.

3. The procedure should be performed in a room well away from the mainstream of theatre traffic.

4. The sources should be transferred to a sterilised lead pot which is placed on a sterile-draped, lead-shielded trolley. Long-handled forceps should be used.

5. A dilation and curettage set should also be prepared.

6. Only the minimum number of staff should remain in the room during the procedure.

7. The patient should be X-rayed before leaving the room to ensure that the sources are correctly positioned.

8. A radiation hazard sign should be placed on the door and also on the trolley used to return the patient to the recovery area and the ward. These patients should be nursed well away from other patients during recovery from anaesthesia.

Afterloading systems

Caesium

In the treatment of carcinoma of the vagina, cervix and uterus, inactive applicators may be inserted in the theatre. An X-ray is taken to ensure that they are correctly positioned. The patient is returned to a single room where special tubes, to accept the radioactive sources, are introduced into the applicators. The sources are then automatically loaded from a storage container. Afterloading systems decrease the risk of radiation hazard to staff and allow the operator more time to ensure that a satisfactory geometrical arrangement has been obtained.

DISPOSABLE MATERIALS

The introduction of disposable material in hospital has brought many advantages, and its use in the operating theatre has allowed nursing staff to devote more time to the care of patients.

The materials generally used for wearing apparel and drapes are paper or non-woven. They should be strong, rustle-free, light in weight and fluid-repellent. Surgical gowns must be tailored for comfort and aseptic protection. Cuffs should be of double-thickness stockinette, and the gown must be designed to cover the wearer's back completely. The manufacturer who produces a pre-sterilised disposable gown which the wearer can tie without the aid of another person will have designed the ideal gown for surgery. Disposable dresses and trousers suits in a variety of man-made fibres are also available for general use.

The wide range of pre-sterilised, fenestrated draping packs available ensures that the fenestration can be correctly positioned in alignment with the surgical site. Areas around the incision site are reinforced to eliminate bacterial migration. Controversy continues as to the cost-effectiveness of using disposable drapes and gowns, but a large proportion of theatres use them for cases where the risk of infection is high. The argument continues that if they are safer for *known* high-risk cases, they should be used as a universal precaution for all surgery in order to achieve the best possible barrier between the patient and the operational field.

The *advantages* of disposable materials are the convenience, the saving of time, and in the case of pre-sterilised packs the assurance of the required standard of sterility. Manufacturers have the advantage of being able to work on a scale which would probably be impossible for a hospital. Disposables are particularly useful during times of staff shortage and also as a reserve when linen supplies are restricted due to laundry problems, industrial action or a breakdown of the hospital sterilising machinery. The fact that they can be delivered from the manufacturer ready for use frees CSSD and theatre staff for other duties.

The possible *disadvantages* of disposable materials are the shortage of materials, the lack of storage space in some hospitals, and the increased use of incinerators for disposal.

A very wide range of disposable equipment is used in the theatre, ranging from nail-brushes and scalpels to drainage material and aerosol cans. Much of the re-usable equipment is sterilised in disposable bags, and all waste material is disposed of in plastic bags. This eliminates the need for handling the material and decreases the risk of infection of staff.

Disposable equipment is now extensively used in anaesthesia. Glass syringes have largely been replaced by plastic and a wide selection of disposable needles are available, but their disposal in the anaesthetic room still remains a problem. The risk of infection from used equipment is ever-present for both patients and staff, and there is a particular need for a safe container for irretrievable disposal of used needles and syringes.

Disposable airways, nasal and oral tubes and intravenous giving sets are of immeasurable value in the operating department.

Disposable and re-cyclable materials

Within the operating department there has been a move in recent years for an increasing number of products to be disposable. This has ranged from surgical drapes to stapling and anastamosis devices. However, as the general public has become aware of environmentally friendly products, so too have theatre staff and product manufacturers.

Increasingly, previously single-use products are now manufactured with certain component for single use and other parts which are re-usable. Bio-degradable properties are now being incorporated into disposable plastics and paper materials. The next wave will certainly see the use of recycled materials to produce a range of products.

FURTHER READING

NATN, *Principles of Safe Practice in the Operating Department: a Resource Book,* NATN, Harrogate, Yorks.

13   Surgical specialities

This chapter will present a brief overview of thoracic, orthopaedic, urological and trauma surgery.

THORACIC SURGERY

A thoracotomy is an incision into the chest wall. The position of the incision depends upon the reason for the surgery. A posterolateral or anterolateral approach, through the ribs, is common in general thoracic surgery. This approach allows the surgeon access to perform a pneumonectomy, lobectomy, wedge resection, thoracoplasty or decortication.

A thoracotomy is classified as a major surgical operation. Competent nursing care of a patient who will have a closed chest drainage system and mechanical ventilation is essential and vital.

Nursing principles

Patients for thoracotomy may have pulmonary conditions such as cancer, benign tumours, bronchiectasis, bullae caused by emphysema or empyema. These patients may have marked respiratory distress prior to surgery and be generally debilitated.

Pre-operative information giving

During the pre-operative phase it is important that these patients are given a general understanding of:

- The purpose of the surgery and the procedures involved.

- The usual surgical scar to expect and knowledge that it will heal to a white line.
- The methods and effects of the anaesthesia.
- The location for recovery in the immediate post-operative period.
- The intravenous fluid therapy lines and other lines which will be attached post-operatively.
- The post-operative oxygen therapy.
- The chest tubes and drainage systems.
- The naso-gastric tubes.
- The use of endotracheal intubation if necessary.
- The effect of the surgery on the lungs and re-expansion methods.
- The amount, nature and methods of control of pain.
- The expected levels of post-operative activity and recovery.
- The use of anti-embolism devices.

In addition to these general requirements, each patient will also have individual knowledge requirements.

Anaesthesia for thoracotomy patients

These patients are given a general anaesthetic and intubated using a double-lumen endobronchial tube. Such a tube enables one lung to be deflated whilst the other is ventilated. In addition, the patients may receive an epidural anaesthetic to assist with post-operative pain. Arterial and central venous pressure monitoring is frequently carried out on patients undergoing a thoracotomy.

The patients are in the lateral position and are well supported on the operating table.

The principles of post-operative patient care

In the immediate post-operative period it is important that the nurse promptly detects any complications. In addition to the normal post-operative care, the nurse must monitor the patient:

For signs of haemorrhage

- which may result from surgical trauma, or inadequate haemostasis. The patient may be tachycardic and hypotensive and have excessive chest drainage.
- decreasing or absent breathing sounds, increasing dull percussion and absent fremitus. This may be due to a haemothorax.
- decreased heart sounds and high central venous pressure. This may be due to a cardiac tamponade.

For signs of a pleural effusion

- decreasing or absent breathing sounds and vocal fremitus. These may be due to a pleural effusion compressing the lungs and causing hypoxaemia.

For signs of a pneumothorax

- Decreasing or absent breathing sounds, dyspnoea and hyperresonance.

For signs of atelectasis

- Fever, tachypnoea, tachycardia, increasing dullness and vocal fremitus. These signs may be due to collapsed alveoli, which produces hypoxaemia.

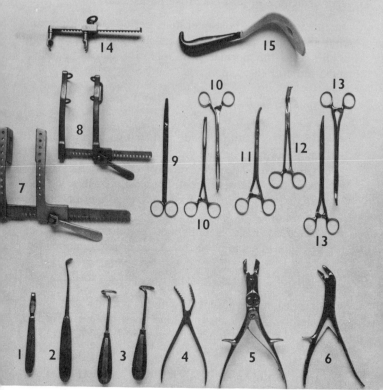

Figure 13.1 Some thoracotomy instruments.

1. Farabeauf's rougine
2. Semb's raspatory
3. Right and left Doyen's rib raspatory
4. Semb's rib-holding forceps
5. Key's compound-action bone cutter
6. Compound action angle rongeurs or nibblers
7. Finochietto's rib spreader with curved scapula blade
8. Ronald Edwards's rib spreader
9. Price Thomas's lobectomy scissors
10. Duval's tissue forceps (2)
11. Price Thomas's pneumonectomy clamp for bronchus
12. Beck's aortic clamp, if needed on pulmonary artery
13. Price Thomas's bronchus clamps (2)
14. Sellor's rib approximator
15. Barrett's lung retractor

For signs of pulmonary oedema

- Tachypnoea, tachycardia, dyspnoea, coughing, wheezing, pink frothy sputum and anxiety.

All of these complications are life-threatening and require medical intervention.

ORTHOPAEDIC SURGERY

The techniques for stabilising fractures have developed over the last decade. In order to introduce the student to orthopaedics, a basic outline of types of fractures and types of fixation will be set out.

Fractures

Open fractures involve tissue damage as well as bone fracture and are usually treated as a surgical emergency. Closed fractures involve bone fractures alone.
  The five most common types of fracture are:

1. *Transverse*. When the fracture is at right angles to the bone shaft.
2. *Spiral*. When the bone fragments rotate around one another and the bone is fragmented.
3. *Comminuted*. When the bone is broken into several components, each a different size.
4. *Impacted*. When one end of the bone is impacted on to the other end.
5. *Oblique*. When the angles of the fracture diverge from the perpendicular axis of the bone.

Fracture reduction

Closed reduction

This involves the external manipulation of the fracture to force it into alignment. Spiral or transverse fractures may be unstable and not suitable for closed reduction.

Open reduction

This method exposes the fracture site by surgical incision and allows the surgeon to re-align the bony fragments by means of internal fixation techniques.

Fixation devices

The use of internal or external fixation devices is determined by the location of the fracture, the type of the fracture and the condition of surrounding tissue.

External fixation devices

These provide rigid immobilisation of the reduced fracture site and include devices such as:

- Casts.
- Splints.
- Continuous traction.
- Skeletal traction.
- Single bar appliances.
- Frame appliances.

Internal fixation devices

These devices are used when an open reduction is performed. A particular device is applied to the bone in order to stabilise it. There are five basic types of internal fixation devices:

Screws. These come in all shapes and sizes and can be used alone or in conjunction with a plate to stabilise a fracture. Screws are either cortical or cancelleous, depending on configuration of the screw thread. Cancelleous bone is soft and will accept a screw without tapping; cortical bone, on the other hand, is hard and requires to be tapped before insertion of the screw. Therefore when using screws it is essential to measure the depth of the screw required, as screws must pass through both types of bone to provide stability.

Plates. These come in a variety of lengths and configuration and can either be tubular or compression in design. A plate stabilises the fracture and provides support for the bone whilst it heals. Plates are usually applied so that there are two screws above the fracture and two below it.

Orthopaedic rods or nails. These are commonly used to stabilise fractures of the middle two-thirds of long bones.

Kirschener wires and Steinmann pins. These are used for the stabilisation of small fractures. They are usually driven into the bone and across the fracture site to provide stability and better alignment of fractured bone ends.

Orthopaedic nail plates. These are used to fixate fractures of the femoral neck and intertrochanteric hip fractures internally.

Tourniquets

Pneumatic tourniquets are frequently used in orthopaedic surgery to compress the limb above the surgical site, thus making the surgical field as free of blood as possible. Care must be taken on application of the tourniquet, as damage can be done to the patient if it is applied incorrectly. Tourniquet timing is important, and most operating departments will have a maximum time limit.

Fractured shaft of femur

This is generally treated by the insertion of a Steinman's or Denham's pin under aseptic conditions and the application of traction.

UROLOGY

In recent years there have been many advances in urological surgery. The most notable was the advent of percutaneous nephrolithrotripsy. Previously, patients who had large renal calculi had to have major surgery performed to remove the stones. This operation often involved a large surgical incision and a long period of recovery.

The development of percutaneous nephrolithrotripsy allows access to the kidney via a percutaneous incision. One method fluoroscopy techniques, a needle is inserted into the calyx of the kidney and aspirated to ensure that urine returns. A guide wire is then passed down the ureter. The tract is usually dilated and the nephroscope inserted, and any blood clots present aspirated with saline. Throughout the procedure saline irrigation continues. An ultrasonic tip is then passed down the nephroscope and this fragments the calculus. If electrohydraulic lithotripsy is required, the flexible nephroscope is inserted and a coaxial electrode is passed down the nephroscope. This electrode touches the stone and fragments it by shock waves. The fragments of the stone are removed either using grasping forceps or by irrigation techniques.

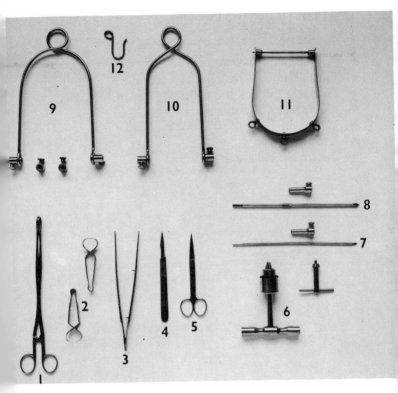

Figure 13.2

1. Sponge-holding forceps
2. Towel clips
3. Non-toothed dissecting forceps
4. No. 3 knife handle with No. 11 blade to make skin excisions for the entry and exit of pin
5. Dressing scissors
6. Handle for introducing pin, with chuck key
7. Steinmann's pin with cap for sharp end
8. Denham's pin (less likely to slip as it has a threaded central portion) with cap
9,10. Böhler's stirrups with adjustment collars (there are three sizes of stirrup)
11. Max Page's stirrup (takes special short pin for fractured calcaneus)
12. Hook connection for cord and traction weights

The instruments required for this surgery include:

- A rigid nephroscope, cystoscope and light source.
- Flexible fibre-optic nephroscopes.
- Grasping forceps and collecting basket.
- Guide wires and dilators.
- Ultrasonic unit.
- Ultrasonic tips.
- electrohydraulic unit and tips.

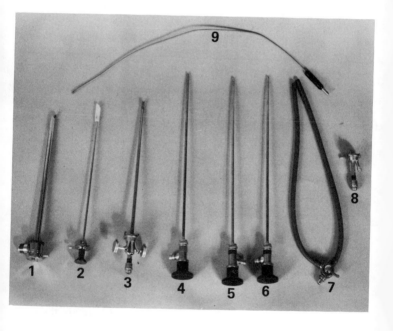

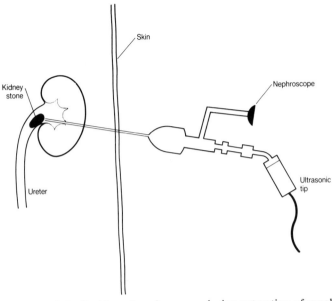

Figure 13.4 Position of nephroscope during extraction of renal calculi.

Figure 13.3 (facing page) Operating cystoscope.

1. Sheath
2. Obturator
3. Catheterising mechanism
4. 0° telescope
5. 30° telescope
6. 70° telescope
7. Water tap
8. Bridge
9. Diathermy electrode

Table 13.1 Some aspects of patient care for percutaneous nephrolithotripsy.

Patient problems	Nursing actions	Outcome
Anxiety due to fear of procedure	Assess patient's anxiety and enable patient to express fear pre-operatively.	Patient communicates anxieties.
Anxiety due to being awake during some of the procedure or due to discomfort	Explain each step before implementation. Maintain calm and quiet environment. Be empathic and supportive. Keep traffic in and out of the room to a minimum.	
Discomfort from low body temperature	Keep room warm. Warm irrigating solutions.	Patient is comfortable.

Potential skin or nerve damage due to positioning.	Transport patient safely. Use radiolucent pad on operating table. Position patient using supports, and secure body alignment. Protect skin from maceration due to pooling of fluids.	No skin breaks, redness or numbness post-operatively.
Potential injury of ureter or kidney by dislodging catheters when transferring patient.	Monitor positioning carefully. Check access to catheters and patency. Secure catheters and drains.	No injury. Catheters patent.
Potential urinary tract infections.	Use aseptic technique to connect catheters. Keep all catheters connected to closed system. Check for gravity drainage, stasis and back flow.	No acute urinary tract infections.

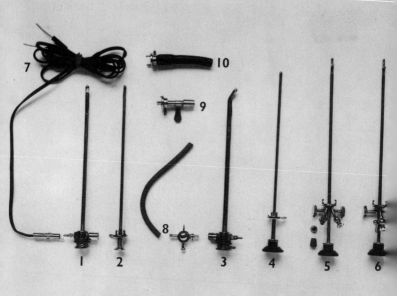

Figure 13.5 Cystoscope.

1. Circular sheath
2. Obturator
3. Oval sheath
4. Examining telescope
5. Double catheterising scope showing Albarran (bridge) raised
6. Single catheterising scope showing Albarran (bridge) raised
7. Light lead (Wappler)
8. Three-way tap and rubber connection
9. One faucet (Thomson-Walker's or Bigelow's)
10. One faucet with rubber tubing for Ellick's evacuator

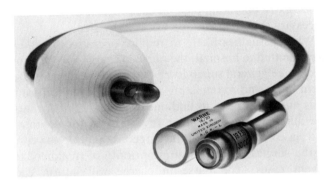

Figure 13.6 Urethral balloon catheter.

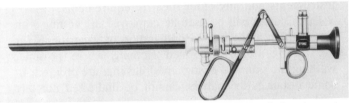

Figure 13.7 Assembled resectoscope in insulated sheath used for transurethral prostatectomy.

TRAUMA

Organisation of theatres

Each hospital will have its own Major Accident Procedure. The operating department plays an important part in any plan for the treatment of large numbers of casualties. Under emergency conditions the theatres will have to work at higher pressure and for longer periods than in normal times; in order to provide for these conditions adequate staff and extra accommodation will be needed. The accommodation problem is usually resolved by setting up an extra operating table in each theatre so that, when necessary, two teams can work side by side.

When casualties likely to require operative treatment are admitted to hospital, the nurse in charge will probably undertake general supervisory duties, assigning an instrument nurse and a circulating nurse to each surgical team. This nurse will need to find out from the accident centre the number and the nature of the cases for operation and, in consultation with the surgeons, allocate the cases to the surgical teams, ensuring priority of treatment for urgent cases. The nurse in charge will inform each instrument nurse of the list for which the nurse will be responsible, and will see that the circulators are given the necessary information so that they may prepare the instruments and any other theatre requirements.

Extra nurses will be usefully employed in assisting with resuscitation and with the preparation of the patients for the theatre, removing soiled clothing where possible, washing the skin and giving any drugs that are ordered. In some instances the patient cannot be undressed nor any preliminary cleansing carried out until he is anaesthetised. The circulator should be prepared to cut off the patient's clothing and should then put it in a labelled bag so that it can be examined later, officially listed and signed into custody. It is important that articles of clothing which may contain important papers or other valuables should not be dropped into soiled dressing buckets and destroyed.

For cutting off clothing, several pairs of stout round-ended scissors of the type sold as upholstery or carpet scissors are very useful. Labels should be provided for clothing bags, and if the patient's name is not known he should be given a number. Small bags are useful for valuables; these should be handed over at once to the person responsible for their safekeeping. If patients who are unconscious or are to be anaesthetised are wearing dentures, these must be removed and placed in a suitable receptacle with the patient's name or number.

Notes made in the accident centre of the patient's injuries and any treatment given, including opiates and tetanus antitoxin given before or on admission to hospital, should accompany the patient to the theatre. If the patient is brought straight from the site of the accident to the anaesthetic room of the theatre, the nurse should look for a label attached to his clothing, or an indelible pencil mark on his person, indicating the suggested diagnosis and the treatment given.

There are various official symbols used in the Emergency Medical Service which should be known to all whose duties include the care of casualties. These are:

'X' The case should receive priority of examination – used for all unconscious cases, suspected internal haemorrhage, and penetrating wounds of the chest and abdomen.

'T' Tourniquet applied; the label should give the time of application and of subsequent releases and reapplications.

'H' The patient has had a severe haemorrhage.

'M' Morphine given; the label should bear the record of the dose and the time at which it was given.

'C' Contamination or suspected contamination with persistent gas, i.e. vesicants.

'XX' Suspected contact with phosgene or other non-persistent gas, i.e. lung irritants.

'P' Phosphorus burns.

Resuscitation and transfusion

In many cases the immediate treatment needed is resuscitation. The theatre staff may have to be responsible for their own equipment; this will include the apparatus for blood and plasma transfusion and stocks of blood, plasma and plasma substitute. Storage of blood and plasma requires a cold store maintaining a temperature between 2.5° and 4.5°C (36°F and 40°F). *Dried* plasma and serum can be kept in any cool dark place. Plasma expanders may also be used.

Double checking must be practised to ensure that the correct blood is given. Failure to do this can endanger life.

When it is necessary to cut down on a vein in order to introduce a needle or cannula, the following instruments should be supplied:

Knife or scalpel
Toothed fine dissecting forceps (1 pair)
Non-toothed fine dissecting forceps (1 pair)
Fine pointed scissors (1 pair)
Fine artery forceps (2 pairs)
Aneurysm needle
Fine thread or catgut
Curved skin needles (2) and sutures
Intravenous cannula, or fine polyethylene tubing with
   adaptor
Syringes, needles and solution for local anaesthesia.

Types of injury

Wounds of the soft tissues

Wounds of the soft tissues may be multiple and may include foreign bodies. The following list of instruments is suggested as representing the basic requirements for dealing with such wounds (including compound fracture, unless amputation is required), i.e. for wound toilet and extraction of foreign bodies.

Towel clips (6)
Sponge-holding forceps (2)
Bard-Parker knives or scalpels
Toothed dissecting forceps, 5-inch and 7-inch
Non-toothed dissecting forceps, 5-inch and 7-inch
Spencer-Wells's artery forceps (12)
Scissors, round-ended and Mayo's
Small and medium retractors
Double hooks
Single hooks
Aneurysm needles
Tissue forceps, Lane's or Allis's (4)
Blunt dissector
Probe
Probe-pointed director
Bone-holding forceps, e.g. Ferguson's lion-jawed
Periosteal elevator
Rugine, e.g. Farabeuf's
Bone-cutting forceps
Needle-holder
Atraumatic sutures
Tulle Gras
Plaster bandages.

When dealing with wounds of the mouth and neck it is necessary to have tracheostomy instruments ready for immediate use.

Compound fractures

All compound fractures are regarded as priority theatre cases. The usual surgical treatment is cleansing of the

limb and excision of the damaged tissue. In some cases
the wound may be sutured. In all cases the limb will be
splinted, usually by plaster, but the theatre nurse should
also have at hand suitably padded wooden splints or
other special splints likely to be used by the surgeon.

Head injuries

Simple scalp wounds are amongst the commonest of
casualties. The preliminary cleaning of the scalp is an
essential step in successful treatment.

The instruments required for dealing with penetrating
wounds of the skull and exploration of an extradural or
subdural haematoma are those used for a craniotomy.

Penetrating wounds of the chest and abdomen

Chest

Operative treatment will probably consist of exploring
the wound, removing damaged tissue and foreign bodies,
drainage, or aspiration and closure. As a basic guide to
the surgeon's requirements the instruments required for
a thoracotomy will normally be used.

Abdomen

Penetrating wounds of the abdomen are urgent emergencies on account of the dangers of general peritonitis
from perforation of hollow viscera and of severe haemorrhage from injury to large blood vessels or such organs
as the liver or spleen. The nurse should enquire if there
is any probability of a colostomy or suprapubic cystostomy
being required, and if there is the nurse should prepare
the appropriate instruments in addition to those needed
for laparotomy.

Burns

In all cases of severe burns, the treatment of shock takes precedence over local treatment. The main cause of shock following burning is the reduction in blood volume due to the escape of fluid from the blood capillaries in the damaged area; the treatment is therefore essentially the replacement of lost fluid by plasma or dextran transfusion.

The patient may be placed on a special frame over which a sterile sheet is stretched, and put into a single air-conditioned cubicle. The area of burns may be left uncovered and sprayed with antibiotic powder to dry up the exudate and form crusts as quickly as possible.

Skin grafting

When loss of skin is extensive, as the result of burns or other injuries, healing is extremely slow and the formation of large areas of scar tissue leads to subsequent contraction, deformity and loss of function. To avoid these results of injury, skin grafting is often carried out as soon as the granulating areas are clean. Occasionally small deep burns, if seen within six hours of the injury occurring, may be excised and grafted without delay.

FURTHER READING

Holloway, N. (1988) *Critical Case Plans*, Springhome Corporation, Pennsylvania.

Glossary of operational terms

Suffixes

Definitions of some of the commoner suffixes may help the nurse to understand strange and often alarmingly long words. However, these word-endings are not always used correctly and in some instances the incorrect terminology is sanctioned by common usage: e.g. the operation of making an opening into the trachea to insert a tube is correctly called a tracheostomy, but is frequently referred to as a 'tracheotomy'. The suffixes '-otomy' and '-ostomy' are the most frequently misused.

-ectomy: a suffix denoting removal or excision of a structure; e.g. hysterectomy (removal of the uterus).

-orrhaphy: a plastic or repair operation; e.g. perineorrhaphy (repair of the perineum). The ending **'-plasty'** is also used, to describe a plastic operation where the aim is to rebuild and restore tissues destroyed by injury or disease.

-oscopy: inspection of the interior of an organ or passage by means of special instruments, usually carrying a light; e.g. cystoscopy (examination of the bladder by means of a cystoscope).

-ostomy: constructing an artificial opening into an organ, e.g. gastrostomy (making an opening from the stomach on to the surface of the abdomen).

-otomy: incising or dividing a structure; e.g. laparotomy (incising and opening the abdomen), tenotomy (dividing a tendon).

Antrostomy. Making an opening into the maxillary antrum to provide drainage. The most extensive type of antrostomy is known as Caldwell-Luc's operation.

Appendicectomy. Removal of the appendix.

Arthrodesis. An operation to stiffen a joint permanently and prevent movement.

Arthroplasty. An operation designed to increase the amount of movement at a joint.

Arthrotomy. Making an opening into a joint for drainage or exploration.

Bronchoscopy. Inspection of the interior of the bronchial tree by means of a bronchoscope. The aspiration of a bronchial abscess, removal of a foreign body or taking a biopsy of a growth may all be carried out as part of a bronchoscopy.

Caesarian section. Removal of the foetus, at or near term, from the uterus by an abdominal incision.

Celsius. To convert degrees Fahrenheit (°F) to degrees celsius (°C) use the formula: $C = \frac{5}{9}(F - 32)$

To convert from °C to °F use: $F = (C \times \frac{9}{5}) + 32$

Cholecystectomy. Removal of the gall-bladder.

Cholecystenterostomy. Establishing an opening between the gall-bladder and the small intestine. Cholecystgastrostomy is a similar operation to connect the gall-bladder and the stomach. These operations are performed to provide drainage of the bile into the alimentary tract when the common bile duct is permanently obstructed, e.g. by the pressure of a growth in the head of the pancreas.

Cholecystotomy. Opening the gall-bladder.

Choledochotomy. Opening the common bile duct.

Chordotomy. Division of nerve tracts within the spinal cord.

Colostomy. Making an opening into the colon to act as a temporary or permanent anus for the discharge of faeces. The usual sites are the descending and transverse colon. 'Caecostomy' is the term used when the opening is made into the caecum.

Colporrhaphy. A repair operation on the vaginal wall in the treatment of pelvic prolapse. Stretching of the anterior vaginal wall and prolapse of the uterus may allow the bladder and urethra to bulge into the vaginal canal, producing the condition known as a 'cystocele', for this the operation of *anterior colporrhaphy* is performed. A similar condition of the posterior vaginal wall, producing a *rectocele*, is dealt with by the operation of *posterior colporrhaphy*. Both these operations may be combined with perineorrhaphy.

Craniotomy. Opening the cavity of the skull, e.g. for the removal of a tumour, to drain an abscess or in the treatment of cranial injuries.

Curettage. Removing tissue by scraping with a curette or spoon. The term is most commonly used for the removal of overgrown lymphatic tissue in the nasopharynx (adenoids), and for curettage of the interior of the uterus.

Cystectomy. Excision of the urinary bladder.

Cystoscopy. Inspection of the interior of the bladder by means of a cystoscope passed per urethra. Catheterisation of the ureters, cauterising papillomata (fulguration) and resection of the prostate gland may be carried out via an operating cystoscope.

Cystostomy. Making an opening into the bladder through

the abdominal wall and inserting a catheter to drain the bladder.

Diathermy. A high-frequency electric current producing great heat. In surgery, diathermy is used for cautery and as a 'diathermy knife' which seals the tissues as it cuts.

Ectopic gestation. Implantation and development of a fertilised ovum outside the cavity of the uterus, usually in a uterine (fallopian) tube. A ruptured ectopic gestation is a condition that usually requires urgent operation.

Embolectomy. Removal of an embolus, or clot, from an artery or vein.

Epididymectomy. Excision of the epididymis, a series of tubules lying behind the testis and continuous with the vas deferens.

Episiotomy. Incision of the perineum in the second stage of labour, to prevent extensive laceration.

Fahrenheit. *See* Celsius.

FG = French Gauge. The Charrière method of marking sizes of catheters; it is the circumference in millimetres.

Gastrectomy. Excision of the stomach. Total removal is an uncommon operation: the usual operation is a partial gastrectomy.

Gastroenterostomy. Making an anastomosis between the stomach and the small intestine, usually the jejunum. Following this operation, the stomach contents bypasses the pyloric end of the stomach and the duodenum; hence the alternative term 'short-circuiting'.

Gastroscopy. Inspection of the mucous lining of the stomach using a flexible gastroscope. Fibrescopes are also used similarly.

Gastrostomy. Making an artificial opening into the stomach for the purpose of feeding a patient with an oesophageal stricture.

Gastrotomy. Opening the stomach for exploration or removal of a foreign body.

Gilliam's operation. An operation for ventro-suspension of retroverted uterus.

Hydrocele. A collection of fluid in the *tunica vaginalis* of the scrotum.

Hysterectomy. Removal of the uterus. A *sub-total hysterectomy* implies removal of the body of the uterus leaving the cervix; *total hysterectomy* is removal of the entire uterus; *pan-hysterectomy* is removal of the uterus, uterine tubes, and ovaries; *radical* or *Wertheim's hysterectomy* is removal of the uterus, appendages, upper part of the vagina and adjacent connective tissue plus pelvic lymph glands.

Ileostomy. Making an opening into the ileum.

Iridectomy. Removal of a section of the iris of the eye as a preliminary to cataract extraction or for the relief of tension in glaucoma.

Jejunostomy. Making an opening into the jejunum.

Laminectomy. Cutting through and removing the laminae of the vertebral column, e.g. in operations for a prolapsed intervertebral disc or as an approach to the spinal cord for removal of a tumour.

Laparotomy. Opening the abdominal cavity. Various conditions which come under the heading of 'acute abdomen' may require an emergency laparotomy, e.g. acute appendicitis, acute cholecystitis, intestinal obstruction (e.g. strangulated hernia, intussusception, malignant growth or volvulus).

Laryngectomy. Removal of the larynx.

Laryngoscopy. Inspection of the interior of the larynx by a mirror and reflected light (indirect laryngoscopy) or by means of a laryngoscope (direct laryngoscopy).

Laryngostomy. Opening the larynx and introducing a laryngostomy tube, an operation sometimes performed in cases of extreme urgency when the glottis is blocked. *N.B.* The terms 'laryngotomy' and 'tracheotomy' are in common use for the operations of introducing a tube into the larynx or trachea, although the correct terms are 'laryngostomy' and 'tracheostomy'.

Leucotomy. Division of some of the white nerve fibres in the frontal area of the brain. The operation is most commonly performed for the relief of mental conditions associated with extreme emotional tension or anxiety.

Lobectomy. Removal of a lobe of the lung.

Manchester repair. Colpoperineorrhaphy, with amputation and reconstruction of the cervix.

Mastectomy. Removal of the breast. 'Radical mastectomy' denotes removal of the breast, the underlying pectoral muscles and adjacent lymph glands in the treatment of carcinoma of the breast.

Meniscectomy. Removal of a cartilage in the knee joint; an operation performed for the condition known as internal derangement of the knee joint (IDK).

Myomectomy. Removal of a fibromyoma or 'fibroid' from the uterus.

Myringotomy. Incision of the tympanic membrane of the ear to drain the middle ear. This operation is also known as *paracentesis tympani*.

Nephrectomy. Removal of a kidney.

Nephropexy. Suturing the kidney to the posterior abdominal wall.

Nephrostomy. Establishing an opening into the pelvis of the kidney for the purpose of drainage.

Nephrotomy. Incising the kidneys, usually for the removal of a renal calculus. This operation is also known as *nephrolithotomy*.

Oesophagoscopy. Examination of the interior of the oesophagus as a diagnostic procedure or for the removal of a foreign body.

Oöphorectomy. Removal of one or both ovaries.

Orchidectomy. Removal of the testis.

Osteotomy. Division of a bone to correct a deformity or as part of an arthroplastic operation. The instrument used is an osteotome and differs from a chisel in that it is bevelled on both sides.

Perineorrhaphy. Repair of the perineum. The term is used for the repair carried out when prolapse of the uterus has occurred as a result of a weakened pelvic floor; it is not usually used for the simple suturing of a lacerated perineum performed immediately after labour.

Pharyngotomy. Opening the pharynx (to gain access to a malignant growth of the upper part of the oesophagus). As the approach is from the side, the operation is known as lateral pharyngotomy.

Pneumonectomy. Removal of one lung in the radical treatment of bronchiectasis, tuberculosis or malignant disease of the lung.

Pneumothorax. A condition in which there is air in the pleural space, with the resulting collapse of the lung.

Prostatectomy. Removal of the prostate gland, which lies at the base of the bladder in the male, usually through a transvesical suprapubic or retropubic incision. Transurethral resection of the prostrate gland is carried out by diathermy or 'cold' punch.

Pyelolithotomy. Removal of a stone from the pelvis of the kidney.

Pyelogram (retrograde). X-ray examination of the renal pelvis after the injection of a radio-opaque medium through a ureteric catheter.

Rammstedt's operation. Incision of the muscular coat of the stomach for the relief of pyloric stenosis in infants.

Splenectomy. Removal of the spleen. Traumatic rupture of the spleen is a common reason for its removal, but the operation may also be performed in certain diseases of the blood.

Tarsorrhaphy. Suturing the eyelids together to protect the eye.

Thoracoscopy. Examination of the pleural space by means of a thoracoscope inserted through the chest wall.

Thoracotomy. Opening the chest cavity, e.g. to drain an empyema or deal with bleeding (haemothorax).

Tracheostomy. Opening the trachea and introducing a tracheostomy tube. In the usual operation, the trachea is opened at the level of the isthmus of the thyroid gland. The operation, referred to as a *high tracheostomy*, may be performed in emergencies, the opening being made through the upper rings of the trachea, which are close to the skin surface.

Trendelenburg's operation. Refers most often to the tying of the internal saphenous vein for varicosed leg veins. Trendelenburg also described pulmonary embolectomy, so that operation is also named after him.

Trephining. Removal of a disc of tissue; usually applied to the removal of a disc of bone from the skull. The term is also used to describe the operation of removing a small disc of the sclerotic coat of the eye in cases of chronic glaucoma.

Ureterolithotomy. The operation of opening the ureter to remove a calculus.

Urethrotomy. Incising the urethra for the relief of stricture.

Index